IBS is BS

A Clear Understanding and Treatment for Your IBS in Layman's Language

LAWRENCE BODNER

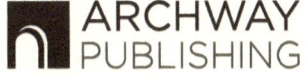

ARCHWAY
PUBLISHING

Archway Publishing books may be ordered through booksellers or by contacting:

Archway Publishing
1663 Liberty Drive
Bloomington, IN 47403
www.archwaypublishing.com
1 (888) 242-5904

ISBN: 978-1-4808-3446-0 (sc)
ISBN: 978-1-4808-3448-4 (hc)
ISBN: 978-1-4808-3447-7 (e)

Library of Congress Control Number: 2016912091

Print information available on the last page.

Archway Publishing rev. date: 08/24/2016

CONTENTS

FOREWORD

Lawrence Bodner offers a wonderful description of his journey from illness to health. Although one might consider this to be a one-off or single-case report, it's personally relevant to the eleven percent of Americans who suffer with Irritable Bowel Syndrome.

While the scientific descriptions and remedies may seem trite, no one else has devised a common-sense language or step-by-step playbook for the over-the-counter treatment of IBS and its ilk.

I have spent my career as a neuropsychiatrist struggling to assess and assist patients with treatment-refractory illness. A fair portion of my patients experience conditions with direct relevance to the topic at hand in this treatise. In order of relative importance to brain disease, I list some common factors here:

- Concussion
- Substance abuse
- Sleep disorders
- Epilepsy and other conditions associated with abnormal EEG
- Adverse effects of medications
- Personality (temperament) factors
- Autoimmune and other immune-based dysfunctions
- Obesity (adipokines)
- Pharmacogenomic adversities

- Nutrition
- Metabolism
- Gastrointestinal infection
- Learning disabilities or giftedness (in particular those children with "regulatory disorders of childhood")
- Tick-borne illnesses
- Environmental poisoning

The gravity of the situation—the avoidable suffering and the impact of GI health on the other portions of the body—should motivate us to carefully consider Mr. Bodner's notions. This book will be a fast read and contains good advice for how a person might choose to help with his or her own health. Neuropsychiatric illness and chronic pain afflict over half of America. It appears that many so-called chronic illnesses (for example hypertension, asthma, diabetes, stroke, and dementia) are also related to diet and gastrointestinal dysfunction.

Helping ourselves means that others don't need to afflict our autonomy—it's liberating for all involved.

Steven Best, M.D.
Neuropsychiatrist

PREFACE

It is often said that everyone has a story to be told, but how many people do, in fact, tell their story? Those who chose to write are usually driven by passion. I equate the art of writing to that of an equation because an equation has two parts: the writer on one side and the potential reader on the other side. So what gives the writer the impetus to write? On the writer's side of the equation, the writer is driven by his or her passion to tell the story bottled up inside his or her brain and psyche. More often than not, the writer's desire to get his or her message or story out is driven by his or her passion to communicate with the public. The reader's side of the equation is his or her desire to educate, entertain, and improve himself or herself and gain knowledge. This book meets all of these criteria.

The subject of irritable bowel syndrome (IBS) is not pleasant, and those people who suffer from this condition certainly do not have a desire to make their condition public. Even though there are in excess of seventy million sufferers in the United States, a fair majority of those members of this detested club suffer in silence.

Part of my character is the possession of the quest for knowledge—particularly in the areas of science and medicine. Human beings who do not have medical issues or illnesses never give them a second thought and often take their lives for granted, living free of pain and unencumbered by illness.

Through my lifelong study of science and medicine, I have been able to deduce a reasonable explanation for IBS and an effective treatment modality. As laymen we have a very warped conception that medicine has all of the answers, but when you look at all of the illnesses and medical conditions that exist without us having a knowledge of a cause or an answer to effect a resolution, then you can grasp the gravity of the situation.

When dealing with experiences of life, we must employee open minds and not always accept the status quo or the pat answer of "that's how it is, and that's what current medicine says it is." The pain, discomfort, and a compromised life of suffering will drive the IBS sufferer to seek all means to achieve a resolution.

ACKNOWLEDGMENTS

I owe endless thanks to my wife and my friends for their encouragement and advice in fostering my drive to get my advisory book into the hands of the general public. My wife, Fran, has always been supportive, and through her diligence, creativity, and culinary attributes she has made my highly restrictive and difficult diet reflect reasonable normalcy and variety. Considering that I have been a type 1 diabetic for forty-seven years, have suffered from IBS for the past fifteen years, and became gluten and lactose intolerant five years ago, my wife, Fran, afforded me a varied and broad diet that circumvented my severe restrictions. Her superior culinary artistic creativity has always afforded me a life of gastronomic pleasures.

In addition, I would like to acknowledge my dear friends who provided me with encouragement to fulfill my dream of getting my IBS message out to help the millions of sufferers of IBS. My dear friend Steven R. Best, MD, a neuropsychiatrist, advised me to go the route of extensive research in order to prove and satisfy my theories. Dr. Best advised against the standard research protocols of double-blind controlled studies because of their prohibitive costs and time involvement. The implications of pharmaceutical intervention and research at this juncture was not an option. During my research, it was Dr. Best who advised me to refer to research and medical publications in veterinary medicine that became of particular importance in my theoretical development.

It was Dr. Best who initially enlightened me about the brain-gut axis and how the role of psychiatric disorders and psychological influences on the body can play a role in irritable bowel syndrome development.

Two additional friends expanded my knowledge and direction in formulating my theories. David Sachs, MD, a friend of mine who is a neurosurgeon, offered me persistent encouragement to pursue writing a book geared to the layman. My dear friend and mentor Thomas A. Sessa, DVM, has always been supportive and invaluable when it comes to theoretical concepts on experimenting with treatment protocols for canine pancreatitis. I am particularly grateful for Dr. Sessa's open weekly invitation to observe surgeries in the OR on Tuesdays; these surgeries encompassed every medical condition and malady. On surgery day I could easily experience fourteen surgeries, depending on the nature of the surgeries and the diagnoses. During surgery and at lunch, I expressed my theories based on the physiological, anatomical, and chemical understanding of IBS and other digestive issues. It was Tommy and other veterinarians who agreed with my hypotheses and said that my theories had efficacy and were amazingly plausible. I owe a great deal to Tommy for his assistance in fulfilling my medical dreams.

A special thanks to my wonderful friend Bobette Wolesensky, who afforded me years of expanded horizons in academia. Her provisions of generosity and inclusiveness at Palm Beach State College, where she had a tenured professorship, provided me with unbridled educational experiences that satiated my thirst for knowledge and empathy. Bobette always supported me and fostered my quests for advancing humanity through empathy. Bobette's unique character of always exuding the quality of giving exemplified her unselfish persona. Her friendship has nourished my soul, and I am forever indebted to her for the gifts she bestowed upon me.

In a final expression of thanks and gratitude, I must acknowledge two PhDs in neuroscience who have published in excess of seventy medical papers on cutting-edge twenty-first-century discoveries in neuroscience and neurology. Robert Spengler, PhD, and Tracey A. Ignatowski, PhD, made groundbreaking discoveries on new delivery routes for treatment medications to the brain. Their work on TNF and anti-TNF agents, along with their discoveries and understanding of neurochemical components (i.e., agonists and antagonists) opened the door to affecting reduction and possible alleviation of pain and suffering from stroke, chronic regional pain syndrome (CRPS), neuropathic pain, traumatic brain injury(TBI), and dementia. Dr. Spengler was initially a professor at medical schools and universities in addition to performing medical research. He discovered that lymphocytes (white blood cells) actually have the ability to communicate with neurons (nerve cells). Robert's patience and guidance in teaching me discipline and proper approach in postulating my theory, as well as his providing me with a clearer understanding of cellular biology and, in particular, neuroscience, were valued assets to me. These doctors' discoveries have broad implications regarding IBS.

Please embark on my eye-opening, insightful tour into the causes and effective treatment resolutions that can help alleviate your suffering. My empathetic goal is to share my knowledge in order to help those who suffer in silence.

INTRODUCTION

If you are reading this, then in all likelihood you are suffering from some degree of irritable bowel syndrome (IBS). If you are not a sufferer of IBS, then chances are you know somebody who does suffer from this malady. There are an estimated seventy million Americans who suffer some degree of IBS. More than likely, you are in the dark as to why you have this malady, have not achieved a resolution or relief, and were never told why you developed this condition.

Statistics can be misleading and inaccurate depending on who did the studies and surveys, and one has to think about how many people suffer in silence. We can further guess how many physicians believe that the etiology, or cause, of IBS can be psychological in origin, discount the patient's complaint, accept it as a natural phenomenon, or do not know how to treat other than referring the patient to a gastroenterologist who might arrive at the same conclusion.

It is my intent that when you read this book, you will have a lot of your questions answered and you will achieve relief and regain a fair degree of normalcy. There is no question that medicine is intimidating to most people, and when a patient is in the presence of a physician, he or she often fails to say to the doctor, "I don't understand what you mean," "What else can I do?" or "Are there other options?" This is a very common scenario that plays out on a daily basis.

In my approach, I will utilize analogies and comparisons to help you understand. Please rest assured that I am not criticizing the practice of medicine. However, I do understand how we got to this current environment. Medicine has radically changed in the last fifty years. The change basically started in 1973 when President Richard Nixon signed into law the Health Maintenance Organization Act on December 29, 1973. This started a series of events that transferred power and medical decision making from the physicians to corporate America. After that, nonmedical lay people employed by medical insurance companies began making medical decisions by acting as gatekeepers in an attempt reduce services in order to curtail the costs incurred by insurance companies while increasing their profits at the expense of the physicians and patients.

You might ask, "What does this have to do with me and my doctor almost forty-five years later?" The answer is that physicians became constrained in their ability to practice medicine. Medicine became corporate-controlled medicine, and the physicians started seeing more patients per day, which reduced the available time a physician could afford to spend on each patient. This simple fact has hurt the physician's ability to practice quality and comprehensive medicine.

The second issue is the advent of computerization, digitization, new modern testing, and an explosion of scientific discoveries. Physicians became reliant on testing and diagnostics, often abandoning their ability to "think outside the box" by being good diagnosticians. Now physicians are forced to answer to government agencies, such as Medicare; corporate entities, such as HMO's; other large medical insurance companies; and possibly large corporate-owned medical practices. The bottom line is that physicians are pressed for time, earn less money than they used to, and are overworked.

The last issue I want to bring up is research. The average person cannot fathom what truly goes into research in terms of money, successful conclusions, and operating under government restrictions and control. Often a patient will balk at the cost of a new medication while asking why he or she pays pennies for a tetracycline tablet and possibly eight dollars or higher for an individual tablet of a newly marketed drug. The answer is that the cost of developing new drugs is astronomical. The success rate of bringing a developing drug to market is somewhere in the 2 percent range. That means that nearly 98 percent of the developing drugs do not make it to FDA approval. These failures are very expensive and damaging to a company's profits. Why the cost? First a pharmaceutical company has to hire scientists and researchers. After they formulate research on a medical condition or disease, they begin to theorize how to correct the condition or disease. Next they utilize chemistry and biology to create a potential drug. The FDA has clear, decisive guidelines and rules to eventually bring a drug to market. A company could easily spend over $2 billion to bring a successful drug to market. It entails first doing animal studies, and if they achieve success, then comes human trial studies, which occur in three phases—not to mention subcategories. In essence, it can take up to ten years and billions of dollars to bring a successful drug to market.

Considering that nearly 20 percent of our population suffers from IBS, it is hard to understand why medicine has not advanced in finding a resolution for IBS. I want you to remember that research started on the animal model, and you will realize why IBS is a possible victim of this premise.

Before we begin, just consider that if you do a Google search on IBS, you will receive 1,400,500 postings. What does that tell you? You will find your answers and solutions as you read this book. Consider this last fact before you become enlightened: the average American eats 1,825 meals and snacks every year. For a person who suffers with IBS, it is just a roll of the dice as to whether that next snack or meal becomes an IBS episode.

Before I begin, I must be emphatic and clear in stating that I am not a licensed physician and I am not diagnosing anyone or promoting a treatment or cure. I am presenting my theory based on recent and past medical research along with my own personal experience in achieving remediation of my IBS.

CHAPTER 1

An Understanding

Part of the IBS problem is how past research has been conducted. The method of how research was modeled and handled hampered the development of an effective diagnosis and correct treatment. In order to understand the potential causes of IBS, I feel the best way to approach this is through six discussions with you. I will approach this by using comparisons of baking a cake and comparing the human body to an automobile, to facilitate easy understanding. These discussions are

- understanding basic human anatomy,
- understanding digestion,
- understanding food contents and components,
- understanding why IBS develops,
- understanding autoimmune disease,
- new concepts and discoveries, and
- treatment protocol.

I shall begin with human anatomy. This discussion will be limited to digestion (i.e., the process by which food is processed by the body, from the mouth to your colon or large intestine). Your body runs on fuel, as you well know, so let's start by looking at the automobile. Please understand that the automobile analogy is only intended for a comparative purpose. We are talking about a gasoline-powered internal-combustion engine here, and the details might not necessarily be relevant to the new cars of today. Your car cannot function and transport you from point A to point B without gasoline to burn to power the engine. When you remove the fuel tank cap and put gasoline into your car, you are providing the food source for your car to produce energy. That gas tank is the mouth of your car. What you put into that tank can affect the efficiency and functioning of your engine.

Think about what can go wrong. You could purchase bad gasoline, low-octane gasoline, or gasoline that has water in it, or you could even purchase diesel fuel by accident. Certainly those substances can affect the efficiency of your engine. Now you must visualize where the gasoline goes when it leaves your tank. Naturally it is transported to your engine via hoses and small pipes. We all know that as an automobile ages, the probability of failures to function properly, efficiently, or at all depends on many different systems that must perform their duties. Gasoline has to be mixed with oxygen and ignited in a chamber to push a piston down to crank a shaft to make your car's wheels move. That's simplistic, but it requires several systems, as you know. Electrical systems energize spark plugs to fire the fuel, water cools the engine, and oil lubricates the moving parts. Yes, it is complex, and when you turn the key to start your engine, you don't give it a second thought.

Don't kid yourself; people pop food into their mouths and don't give it a thought after it passes their taste buds in their mouths and fills their stomachs. My purpose for giving you the automobile analogy is that it is fairly easy to understand and visualize. When you think about it, your digestive system is quite similar in intent and purpose.

Just as an automobile has a fuel pump, a battery, an alternator, an oil pump, a radiator, and other parts, your digestive system has many complex parts and systems too. I might be presenting an awful lot of information here, but if you don't understand the basics of metabolism and anatomical function, then you cannot understand your IBS, its causes, and its methods of treatment.

There is an old saying—"Know thy enemy!" It is often said that if you don't know and understand your enemy, then you can never win the war—and this battle is a war.

Let us start by eating a meal. It is lunchtime, and you are planning to eat a ham sandwich on white bread with Swiss cheese and butter, a handful of cherries, a peach, and a dish of ice cream for dessert. After lunch you still want something sweet, but you feel guilty, so you eat a sugar-free chocolate bar that has almonds and contains mannitol, sorbitol, and maltose.

The unfortunate thing is that you have IBS. What happens after twenty minutes, one hour, two hours, and how do you feel the next morning? You may experience sharp abdominal pain, gas, bloating, cramping, loose stools, and frequent bowel movements.

Imagine you were invited to dinner at someone's home and he or she made an elaborate dinner for eight people. The table was elaborately set, and there were appetizers and drinks in the living room. On the coffee table were a variety of cheeses, nuts of all kinds, spicy Indian food samplings, dips, crackers, and peach daiquiris.

An hour later, you were invited to the dinner table to begin the feast. First, shrimp cocktail was served with heavy spicy tomato sauce, followed by a salad with a creamy dressing on lettuce, tomatoes, avocados, mozzarella cheese, onions, dried cherries, and almonds. The main course arrived after that, consisting of fish that was sautéed in butter and had a cheese topping with garlic cloves.

Needless to say, I know how you felt the next day. An estimated 20 percent of the American population suffers from IBS. The scenario I portrayed does not fit everyone, and this is the perplexing problem of this disorder. I will explain why it does not present clearly and equally, why there are varying degrees of IBS, and why it can be intermittent.

Now for the journey. Just as the gasoline in your car moves from the tank (your car's mouth), your food follows a similar path. In your mouth, your saliva moistens and lubricates the food to prepare your food for the journey. Your saliva also contains amylase, an enzyme produced by your salivary glands that breaks down starch into simpler sugars such as maltose. Digestion and metabolism is a long, slow, and complex series of processes and events.

You read labels on food packages so you can clearly see the ingredients. We are all aware of the three basic components of food (i.e., fats, proteins, and carbohydrates). Amylase is an enzyme, and the function of an enzyme is to act as a catalyst. What that means is that it starts a chemical reaction and helps accelerate the reaction but does not become part of the reaction. The chemical reaction breaks down the starch into other smaller molecules and simpler components.

Now back to our car's complex system that converts fuel into energy. As intimidating as mechanics can be when discussing your car, you are basically dealing with one type of fuel—gasoline. The human body's complexities are influenced by well over twenty-six different enzymes that are produced in your mouth, stomach, pancreas, and small intestine, along with countless fuel sources—namely your varied diet's different foods.

I wish I could apologize for the complexities of human digestion, but it is necessary to understand it in order for you to realize why you have IBS, what causes it, and what actually is the condition called IBS.

After your food leaves your mouth (your car's gas tank), the complexities and roadblocks start their war of havoc. If you are a chemist, have an understanding of chemistry, or have a background in chemistry, then you are in luck and have an advantage over most of us. For those of you who are bakers and chefs, you have an advantage too. Your advantage is that you might even unconsciously have a working knowledge of chemistry and physics. Just think about that for a moment. What is entailed in baking a cake, bread, pastries, soufflés, and other complex dishes? What are the variables that the baker encounters during the entire baking process? You have to worry about temperature, timing, barometric pressure, humidity, duration of baking, and the ingredients.

Baking is a chemical process, and catalysts are used to start the process. Just think about the complexities of the art of baking. The baker has to understand quantities of ingredients, ambient temperature, ingredients, humidity, oven temperature, duration of cooking, and the timing involved in adding each ingredient to the batter. (By the way, the food in your stomach is called chyme and is, in essence, the batter in the digestion process.)

Now for the fun. Back to your car. Do you live in North Dakota in January? Do you live in South Florida in August? Just think about how temperature and humidity can affect your car. Have you ever had trouble starting your car? Try to remember why you had trouble. If it was -20 degrees F, did you have starting issues? Were you in a deep freeze for ten days straight? Did ten days straight of temperatures in the high nineties, 100 percent humidity, frequent rain, and flooding ever affect your car?

You can understand that certain environmental conditions affect your car's engine's ability to perform. Don't think for a second that your body's environment does not affect your digestive process. It is time to drop the bomb. Just as we briefly touched on your car's mouth, the gas tank, and your car's stomach, the engine, it is time to get to the core of what variables affect your IBS.

In your car's engine, digestion begins. Of course that is a metaphor, but what I mean is that your car's engine goes through a process of mixing the gasoline with oxygen and igniting it with an electric spark. This all occurs in a chamber, the cylinder, which is comparable to your stomach. Now we must discuss what happens in your stomach. Your stomach produces six enzymes that are responsible for the early phase of digestion. Remember: when you make the batter for a cake, you mix the ingredients. Well, your stomach performs this same function, churning and mixing its contents. The length of time that food (chyme) remains in your stomach is a wild guess because of the many variables involved, but generally speaking, it is from two to five hours. The variables are the amount of food, the type of food, and other factors about the individual.

The human body is the most amazing and complex machine that was ever created. It is important to understand that the human body has a dual chemical manufacturing plant on board that is an active part of your digestive system. This important organ is your pancreas, which is shaped like a large carrot and is located behind the stomach, adjacent to the liver and intestines. I call the pancreas a dual manufacturing plant. It produces the enzymes responsible for the start of the process of digesting fats, proteins, and carbohydrates. I call it a dual manufacturing plant because it serves two separate functions. Just 1 percent of the organ is responsible for the production of insulin. This function of the organ is called the endocrine function of the pancreas, and that means that the insulin it manufactures is dumped directly into your bloodstream. Insulin is responsible for facilitating the movement of the glucose from your bloodstream into your individual cells. Glucose is the fuel that every cell in your body runs on. When the beta cells in your endocrine pancreas, which are located in the islets of Langerhans (small island-like structures throughout 1% of the pancreas) are compromised, no longer function, and die, then you become a type 1 diabetic.

A type 1 diabetic has no more beta cells, can't produce anymore insulin, and will die without replacing that insulin via injections of replacement insulin. Type 2 diabetes is due to either reduced insulin production because of a reduction in the population of beta cells in the person's pancreas, or insulin resistance, which prevents insulin from ferrying glucose into the body's cells. Obesity is a major cause of type 2 diabetes because the excess tissue cannot be serviced by the limited amount of insulin produced or because of increased insulin resistance.

Now for the other twin of this manufacturing plant. This is called the exocrine function of this organ. This means that the other 99 percent of the pancreas produces enzymes, which number nine in total. These enzymes are for the main digestion process, and they are dumped directly into the duodenum via a pancreatic duct. The duodenum is the first section of your small intestine, which food enters right after leaving your stomach.

CHAPTER 2

The Majority of the Rest of Your Pancreas

Trust me; I do not wish to lecture you or overwhelm you with information, but there is no shortcut to correcting your IBS issues. Think for a moment. Would you attempt to bake a complex cake without knowing what ingredients to have on hand to add, when to add the yeast, whether or not to preheat the oven, how long to bake it, and at what temperature to bake it?

Put on your seatbelt, and let's take a trip to your stomach, pancreas, and small intestine. Everybody is aware that our stomachs are acidic. How many people use antacids and suffer from hyperacidity (elevated levels of stomach acid)? It's not pleasant and certainly makes sufferers feel lousy because of the resultant pain and burning. This is an extremely important consideration in the digestion process and an absolute consideration when food enters one's duodenum. How many medications have you taken that bear the warning "take with food" or "take on a full stomach"?

As a side note, just ask yourself if your doctor ever discussed with you the intricacies and variables that are encountered during the whole digestive process. I am now prepared to show you a list of what I have been talking about since you started reading this book. Please do not be shocked, overwhelmed, or hung up on this information now, because we will gradually delve into each item on the surface as we get to each stage of digestion. Remember that every person who receives a diagnosis of irritable bowel syndrome does not present with exactly the same symptoms at the same intensity. You will soon realize why some people have so-called mild symptoms and infrequency, as opposed to others, who present with severe symptoms on a daily basis.

Here is what we are dealing with:

Mouth Enzymes
1. Ptyalin—converts starch to simple soluble sugars
2. Amylase—converts starch to soluble sugars
3. Betaine—maintains cell fluid balance as osmolytes
4. Bromelain—anti-inflammatory agent, tenderizes meat

Stomach Enzymes
1. Pepsin is the main gastric enzyme. It breaks proteins into smaller peptide fragments.
2. Gelatinase degrades type I and type V gelatin and types IV and V collagen, which are proteoglycans in meat.
3. Gastric amylase degrades starch but is of minor significance.
4. Gastric lipase is a tributyrase by its biochemical activity, as it acts almost exclusively on tributyrin, a butterfat enzyme.
5. Pepsin, an enzyme, is secreted by gastric glands and aids in protein breakdown.
6. Renin, an enzyme, changes liquid milk to a solid.

Pancreas Enzymes
1. Pancreatic lipase—degrades triglycerides into fatty acids and glycerol (fat breakdown).
2. Chymotrypsin—converts proteins to aromatic amino acids
3. Carboxypeptidase—degrades proteins to amino acids
4. Pancreatic amylase—degrades carbohydrates to simple sugars

5. Elastases—degrades the protein elastin
6. Nucleases—converts nucleic acids to nucleotides and nucleosides
7. Trypsin—converts proteins to basic amino acids
8. Steapsin—breaks down triglycerides to glycerol and fatty acids
9. Phospholipase—hydrolyzes phospholipids into fatty acids and lipophilic substances

Small Intestine Chemicals (Brush Border Cells)
1. Cholecystokinin—a hormone that stimulates digestion of proteins and fats
2. Secretin—a hormone that promotes secretion into the duodenum and osmoregulation
3. Sucrase—converts sucrose to disaccharides and monosaccharides
4. Maltase—converts maltose to glucose
5. Lactase—converts lactose to glucose and galactose
6. Isomaltase—converts maltose to isomaltose
    Wikipedia - Thomas A. Brown "Rapid Review Physiology" Mosby Elsevier, 1ˢᵗ Ed. P. 244}

I know what you are saying right now: "It's all Greek; why do I need to even look at this?" You do not need to remember all of this or understand the chemical nature of each enzyme, but I want you to be aware of the fact that each component or ingredient of food needs a specific enzyme (i.e., a catalyst) to start the chemical reactions that break down the food so your body can utilize it.

Now for the bombshell. How did medicine and science go wrong by calling your condition IBS? Just take a peek at the list above. Think about the fact that if you are deficient in one or more of the above enzymes, then what would be the end result? IBS, of course!

Ah, so your doctor told you that you have IBS. What does that mean? Does that mean that your doctor is telling you, "Well, your symptoms of gas, bloating, pain, cramps, frequency of bowel movements, soreness, and soft stools are the result of a condition we call IBS"? This is what is irritating, frustrating, and not fair. Were you told the cause of your IBS? Were you ever told how it can be treated? Did your doctor ever explain to you about the complexities of digestion or the possibility of becoming deficient in any one of the enzymes listed on the chart on the previous page?

It is time to understand the process we call digestion. When you ingest a food and it enters your mouth, you begin to chew. This breaks down the food into smaller pieces and mixes it with the saliva to lubricate it and predigest it to some degree, depending on its composition. If it's a starch, then the amylase in your saliva starts to assist in breaking down the starch into sugar. The ptyaln converts the sugars into simple sugars. It is extremely rare that there would be any known dangers to you at this stage.

The next stop is your stomach, and now we can encounter our first stressor or roadblock—stomach acid. This acid is called hydrochloric acid, which is a very powerful acid and can be the cause of many issues. At this point you have already been exposed to ten enzymes (four in your mouth and six in your stomach). That leaves us with sixteen more to consider (nine enzymes from your pancreas and four from your small intestine).

Remember when you baked your first cake. Did you preheat the oven and by chance forget to lower or raise the temperature when you put the batter into the oven? If you baked from scratch, did you ever forget to add the yeast? Did you ever forget baking soda, baking powder, or cream of tartar if required? Well, unfortunately, similar situations occur in IBS, except it's not that your body forgets the ingredients.

Rather, your body fails to produce some of those enzymes that aid in breaking down the ingredients in the batter, your stomach contents.

If you look at the chart on the previous page and check out the enzymes produced in your stomach, you will realize that fat metabolism begins there. There is some degree of milk digestion in the stomach, as renin converts liquid milk into a solid, but milk sugar digestion does not really occur until the chyme reaches your small intestine, specifically your ilium, the last section of your small intestine. I am jumping the gun here, but lactose intolerance is caused by your inability to produce the enzyme lactase, which breaks down the lactose (milk sugar) molecule. The enzyme lactase is produced mainly in your jejunum and ilium by your brush border cells. I will discuss this later.

As the title of the next chapter says, you are at ground zero. Of course you realize why I use the baking and automobile analogies to ease you into understanding why medicine named the condition IBS. As we all know, life is not perfect. Depending on how many years you own your car, there are no guarantees that the engine will always start when you turn the key, the air conditioning will always work, or the transmission will always function normally. The same goes for baking. If you bake from scratch and you use very old yeast that becomes inactive, the possibility of your bread or cake not rising is quite real. Ingredients, timing, and temperature are all essential considerations. Keep that in mind, and you will understand the minefields that you will encounter in the duodenum and the rest of your small intestine. If you observe the percentages, you can get a feel of the complexities that arise at this stage of digestion. Remember that the stomach sees only 11.5 percent of the action.

CHAPTER 3

Ground Zero for IBS

Based on my own research and my discussions with veterinarians and a medical researcher, I figured out why medicine missed the cause of IBS. Earlier in this book I discussed how the practice of medicine has changed. Concerning the cost of prescription pharmaceuticals, I explained why new drugs that come on the market cost so much. Remember the part about using animal models? Well, that's the key.

In order to understand what I am talking about, we should first look at the medical condition called pancreatitis. Pancreatitis can be acute or chronic. In the acute form, it is a one-time ailment that causes inflammation of the pancreas that eventually resolves, and the organ returns to normal with few or no aftereffects, depending upon the severity of the infection. The chronic form of pancreatitis is, in essence, a reoccurring inflammation. In the chronic form, the patient suffers the after-effects throughout life. What are these after-effects? In essence they are the compromised ability of the organ to produce some of the exocrine pancreatic enzymes necessary for digestion. Remember that your pancreas produces nine enzymes, and one or more might become insufficient or deficient as a result of pancreatic ailments.

This is the exact turning point at which medicine made a huge error. A physician who suspects a patient is presenting with pancreatitis will order a CAT scan and possibly an ultrasound of the pancreas. In addition, a blood test will be performed to measure serum lipase and amylase enzymes in the blood. Finally he or she will order a special elastase stool test (El1) to determine whether there is fat in the stool sample, which would indicate deficient fat digestion. If these return as positive, then the diagnosis is more than likely pancreatitis. Think about this for a moment. How did medicine end up being so concentrated on the lipase enzyme, which breaks down fat, and amylase, which helps metabolize starches? The answer is the canine. Yes, dogs were studied extensively, and after studies and controlled experiments, scientists determined that if a patient is deficient in lipase and amylase after an ailment of the pancreas (pancreatitis), the inflammation is the cause. This scenario likely arose from the research and experimentation that Banting and Best performed on canines that eventually led to their discovery of insulin and the treatment for type 1 diabetes. This was done during the second decade of the twentieth century and culminated in their insulin discovery in 1921.

Can one use the canine model to understand and diagnose the human? Well, scientists said that since canines are mammals with the same basic anatomy and digestive system as humans, this can work. I say it can't, because what they left out was diet. If you are attempting to understand IBS, then this is where the trouble arises. IBS means "I don't know what is wrong with you." If your lab tests prove negative, then the physician assumes you don't have chronic pancreatitis and you must have IBS. "But I don't know what causes it," the physician often answers.

I am discussing three of the nine pancreatic enzymes out of all digestive enzymes. The reason the researchers singled out amylase and lipase is because of the canine diet. What do dogs eat? Meat, of course, and when you realize that dogs eat the same food day in and day out without variation, you can see the flaw in their studies. Do the math; three out of nine enzymes were studied, meaning that the researchers concentrated on only 11.5 percent of all of the digestive enzymes. If you want to understand IBS, then study the human diet and not the canine diet. Let us compare the average dog to the average American person. Does your dog have a steady diet of fruits, particularly peaches, cherries, blackberries, and juices, along with beans, cheeses, milk, ice cream, avocados, garlic, onions, and candies laden with sugar, mannitol, sorbitol, or maltose? I can go on and on about this.

So what is the lesson here? The truth is that current medicine is hung up on just 11.5 percent of the potential problem and etiology of IBS. Deductive reasoning should be employed here. In the chapter on diagnosis and treatment, I will show you how to institute this tool to help you and your doctor arrive at your specific diagnosis and form of treatment.

At this stage, you are likely more than anxious to find out the root cause of IBS. What is amazing is that the answer is simple in theory but complex in relation to the subtypes of IBS. By this I mean that IBS is a general term for many specific conditions that can develop in one or more of the five regions of your digestive system—your mouth, stomach, pancreas, small intestine (duodenum, jejunum, ilium), and large intestine.

Now turn on your GPS and see where we are now. To refresh your memory, we are still in your car's engine, your stomach. Here is another consideration to address—the length of time the food remains in your stomach. The time can vary from two hours and range up to five hours; estimates vary from publication to publication. As you read this book, I will keep reiterating the importance of the pH (degree of acidity or alkalinity) in your digestive system—particularly your stomach and small intestine.

What goes on in the stomach? Think of your stomach as your bowl and electric mixer that you use to turn your cake ingredients into batter. The stomach's muscles work on churning and reducing the chyme into smaller pieces, moistening it, and adding into the mix, gastric juices and stomach acid (hydrochloric acid with a low pH). Renin is also released to change liquid milk into a solid. With these three main stomach enzymes present, the starches, fats, and proteins start to become reduced into smaller molecules that are broken-up components of the larger starch, fat, and protein molecules. If you have hyperacidity (high hydrochloric stomach acid), then many problems can arise. Some of them you are likely very familiar with; they can include acid reflux, indigestion, a burning feeling, soreness, and even abdominal pain. There is also another issue that can arise; a highly acidic stomach environment can destroy or reduce the effectiveness of supplemental enzymes that you might take.

This is the first consideration in the quest to understand and treat IBS. To make it easy to understand, consider your car. If you have a gasoline engine in your car and you feed it diesel fuel, what happens? No go! Just as you can't burn diesel fuel in a gasoline engine, you can't break down food components in the chyme without the proper active digestive enzymes present.

If you take a peek at your GPS, you will note that we are leaving the stomach after being here a few hours, and we are entering the first section of the small intestine. It is important to look around and view your GPS map carefully. The surroundings are very different here in your duodenum. The topography is quite different than that of your stomach lining. The first thing you will notice here is the very hilly landscape as opposed to the folds of the stomach lining. You can see fingerlike projections called villi. The word *villi* is from Latin, meaning "tufts of shaggy hair." In addition, the lining is called the mucosa, and yes, it does have a mucus-like film over it, which serves many purposes, but the main one is protection and lubrication. All throughout your entire digestive tract are multiple types of bacteria. The human digestive system actually has ten trillion resident bacteria comprising one thousand species. This mucosal lining helps prevent these bacteria from migrating or entering into other parts of your body and keeps them corralled in the intestines. The mucosa also helps the chyme move easier through the intestines. Your intestines also have sheets of muscles that create movement to carry the food through the intestines.

If you stop to check the weather (pH) here, you will note that a radical change occurred as you entered the duodenum. The environment went from an acidic environment in the stomach (a pH of 2.2–3.3) to a basic environment. This is accomplished by the production of sodium bicarbonate in the pancreas. The function of this action is to convert the chyme from an acidic mass in the stomach to a basic or alkaline mass that will be prepared to receive the pancreatic and duodenal (brush border) enzymes in the duodenum. This is of utmost importance in understanding IBS.

My purpose in presenting detail and intricacy here is to provide you with a broad overview of the complexities of digestion. Your concentration and understanding purely depend upon your desire to stop the suffering you sustain from IBS. All too often, Americans believe that there will always be a little pill to correct a medical malady or a corrective procedure to repair a damaged region or organ. Sorry, but as you read, you will understand why those simple solutions are not the answer here. However, don't despair, because I will offer you treatment that works.

Looking at the material covered to date, it would be a good time to review the pH values of common solutions that you are familiar with. A pH reading can range from 0.00 to 14.00. Zero, for example, is battery acid and is the most acidic; while lye, at fourteen, is the most basic. Water is neutral at 7.00. Here are some common examples of solutions you know:

Solution	pH Value	
battery acid	1.00	(extremely acidic)
sulfuric acid	1.00	
lemon juice, vinegar	2.00	
Orange juice, soda	3.00	
tomato juice	4.00	
black coffee	5.00	
milk, urine	6.00	
pure water	7.00	(neutral)
human blood	7.40	
eggs, seawater	8.00	
baking soda	9.00	
milk of magnesia	10.00	
ammonia	11.00	
bleach	12.00	
oven cleaner	13.00	
caustic soda	13.5	(extremely alkaline)

Naturally, you are thinking, *Why the importance and consideration of pH?* This is the most important consideration in proper digestion and digestive function alongside the necessity of the enzymes required to facilitate the normal digestive process, because an acidic environment can destroy enzymes.

It is clear that pH values are extremely important in the human body. The stomach has been covered, and for a quick review, your stomach is like a bowl and an electric mixer used in baking. Your stomach is responsible for approximately 10 percent of your digestion. At the top part of your stomach the pH could be in the 4.0–4.5 range, and as you travel lower, the pH can drop to 2.5. Basically your stomach performs pre-digestion, and that's why I compare it to making the batter in baking. The stomach mixes and grinds the food (chyme) with stomach acid, amylase, renin, and protease. This starts the pre-digestion process.

Now back to our current location—the duodenum. This is where the majority of action takes place. Approximately 90 percent of the digestive process occurs in the small intestine, and a majority of that occurs in the duodenum. In general, absorption takes place in all three sections of the small intestine. That means that your body derives its energy and sustenance from here. It is time to turn on your GPS and look at your surroundings. The chyme from the stomach enters the duodenum through the pyloric valve in small amounts about every twenty seconds and is bathed in a secretion having a pH of 6.0–8.5. This is ground zero for IBS. If there is something that can go wrong with the digestive process, it more than likely occurs here. If you look at the wall of the duodenum, you will notice an opening or hole from a duct that is attached to the duodenal wall. This duct transports the exocrine enzymes from your pancreas to the duodenum to commence the chief digestion process. Bear in mind that along with those pancreatic enzymes, the intestinal enzymes, known as the brush border enzymes, play a major role in digestion too.

Now you can understand why pH is so important. Remember that a low pH will destroy the exocrine pancreatic enzymes and intestinal enzymes. Therefore, your pancreas actually produces sodium bicarbonate, and it travels via the duct from the pancreas to the duodenum. This prepares the environment in the duodenum by gradually increasing the pH to 6.0–8.5 in order to prevent the destruction of pancreatic and intestinal enzymes. Also, bile produced in the liver comes from the gallbladder via the pancreatic duct and is dumped into the duodenum for stabilization of fats and aid in their absorption.

Since 90 percent of digestion occurs in the small intestine, that is why I call it ground zero. Three key enzymes produced in the pancreas—amylase, lipase, and trypsin—enter the duodenum via the duct connecting the two and are ready to help further break down proteins, fats, and carbohydrates after initial action in the stomach.

There is one last and most important geographical observation to be made here. Remember those guys called villi, the fingerlike mountainous structures that protrude into the duodenum? Well, put on your seatbelt, because this is the key to IBS. You will now find out something shocking that no one ever told you about IBS, and that is the actual cause.

These microvilli are on your brush border cells (enterocytes). This, I believe, is where the problems that are responsible for IBS arise. The glandular cells dispersed in the brush border manufacture six key enzymes responsible for the digestion of a fair majority of your diet besides the meats, starches, and fats. Remember this chart?

Small Intestine Enzymes (Brush Border Cells)
1. Cholecystokinin—a hormone that stimulates digestion of proteins and fats
2. Secretin—a hormone that promotes secretions into the duodenum and osmoregulation
3. Sucrase—converts sucrose to disaccharides and monosaccharides

4. Maltase—converts maltose to glucose
5. Lactase—converts lactose to glucose and galactose
6. Isomaltase—converts maltose to isomaltose
    Wikipedia - Thomas A. Brown "Rapid Review Physiology"
    Mosby Elsevier, 1ˢᵗ Ed. P. 244}

Now for the amazing discovery. I want you to think about all of the foods that you eat beside meat, potatoes, and fats. Think of your symptoms (e.g., gas, bloating, cramps, soft stools, and frequent bowel movements). Why do these things this happen, and why do you have these feelings? The answer lies right where you are now in your digestive journey.

Just look at those six enzymes and see what they do. Just imagine what would occur if your brush border cells could not produce the enzymes they are supposed to make. Eureka—you get IBS. It is important to note that the lining of your intestines, where the villi protrude into the intestine, is called the mucosa, and its functions are protection and lubrication.

Next I will identify the brush border cell enzymes and explain their functions. Cholecystokinin stimulates the digestion of protein and fats. Secretin controls all of the secretions and osmoregulation of the duodenum. This is very important, because if your ability to produce secretin is compromised, then the production of the duodenal enzymes could be hindered, and if you can't control osmosis in your duodenum, it can affect your stool. Osmotic regulation is the control of fluids (water) across the wall of your small intestine. Ever hear of the medical term "leaky gut"? In addition to excessive gluten ingestion, low production of secretin can affect digestion.

Now for the other four duodenal brush border enzymes. If you cannot produce these enzymes, or if you do not produce enough enzymes, then you will experience every symptom of IBS and you might even develop small intestinal bacterial overgrowth (SIBO). The reason for this is that sucrase, maltase, lactase, and isomaltase are responsible for breaking down sugars. Sugars come in many varieties and types. Sugar is a general term, and examples are milk sugar (lactose) fruit sugar (fructose), glucose, maltose, and others. These sugars are large, complex molecules that need to be broken down for the body to be able to utilize their components.

Just think about what happens if you don't produce these enzymes to break down these large, complex sugar molecules into smaller molecules and products that your body can use. The easiest way to understand why the failure to break down these sugars results in IBS and possibly SIBO is to just look at brewing beer or baking a cake or bread. The key is fermentation. When you use yeast—which is an active organism, a fungus—to make bread rise, it converts sugar into alcohol, carbon dioxide, and possibly hydrogen gas. (That is why you add sugar to yeast in order to stimulate yeast reproduction and fermentation action.)

Realize that your duodenum and your entire intestines are laden with naturally occurring bacteria. Normally the resident bacteria maintain an average population, but what would happen if the bacteria were to encounter a smorgasbord of assorted sugars? They would go wild and multiply like crazy. In essence, these bacteria are fermenting these sugars. Just as in fermenting beer, your duodenum and intestines in general are filling up with gas from the fermentation. This in turn produces cramping and bloating. Soft stools result, and frequent bowel movements prevail; I will discuss the cause of this shortly.

And where do these sugars come from? This simple question explains why medical research on IBS and pancreatitis is flawed. Remember that researchers used the canine animal model for their studies. How many of you have ever had a dog as a member of your family? Think of your dog's lifestyle and habits. I am talking about your friend's canine diet. The average person does not have a clue what occurs in the dog food industry, and I am not discussing ethics here. What I am discussing is the engineering and manufacturing of dog food that we call kibble, as well as a lot of canned dog food. These foods are engineered and formulated for the masters of the dogs. These companies have actually studied and formulated foods based on the digestive processes that occur in dogs. These so called "modern" foods were formulated to metabolize slowly for the benefit of the dog's master in order to reduce the dog's necessity for relieving himself. These foods were actually engineered for the human lifestyle, (i.e., people being gone all day while their dogs stay at home alone).

When kibble is manufactured, it is baked at high temperatures. It contains a large quantity of salt and is dried in ovens at high temperatures. Hence, dogs become quite thirsty after eating the kibble. After ingestion, the kibble expands in their stomachs by reconstituting itself or hydrating by absorbing water. If you doubt that, then just take a piece of kibble and drop it into a glass of water and observe. I am telling you this for a few reasons. The chief reason is that the canine diet is a far cry from our diets, and therefore, when canines were used in animal studies for understanding pancreatitis and possibly IBS, the researchers failed to take into account the diet variations between that of the canine and that of the human. Just realize that dogs do not have the same human diet of all of the various sugar-containing foods.

As I said, the duodenum is ground zero, and since 90 percent of the digestion and absorption of nutrients occurs in the small intestine, particularly the duodenum, we should look at why I believe this is ground zero for IBS. You have traveled through the mouth, stomach, and pancreas, and have now made it to the duodenum. The easiest way to understand my theory on the etiology of IBS is to read about and understand the FODMAP diet.

A recent development in the treatment of IBS is to follow a FODMAP diet. So what is a FODMAP? "FODMAP" is an acronym that stands for "fermentable oligiosaccharides, disaccharides, monosaccharides, and polyols." What do you see there? You see all of the bad guys for someone who suffers from IBS. These FODMAPs are the complex sugars IBS sufferers can't break down into smaller molecules because they no longer produce the enzymes, or lack enough enzymes, for digestion.

In order to understand IBS, a physician, patient, or layman must truly understand what actually occurs at this stage of digestion and understand all of the components and ingredients of food. A little later I will explain my theory of why people develop IBS and its etiology.

Remember that if you can't metabolize or break down these complex sugars, you are leaving all of these sugars available to your resident bacteria. If this repeatedly occurs, you are setting yourself up for the possible development of SIBO. Just think about the fact that without the ability to digest or break down these complex sugars, you are in essence setting up a brewery in your duodenum, the first section of your small intestine. Just as you add yeast to brew beer or bake a cake or bread, you are doing the same in your digestive tract. When you use those little yeast animals (fungi) to make cakes and bread rise, they feed on the sugar you added to the batter, and they multiply and break down the sugar into alcohol and carbon dioxide gas. That gas that makes the bread rise, the cake rise, and the beer ferment also does the same to the chyme containing FODMAPs.

Please realize that fermentation is not only caused by or initiated by yeast. Many bacteria accomplish the same thing and are utilized in the production of specific products, such as vinegar and sourdough bread. It is hard to believe, but you are accomplishing the same thing in your duodenum, jejunum, and ilium.

Now it is time to find out where these complex sugars come from. When you look at that acronym, the conglomerate of six different sugars, you must say to yourself, "What foods contain them?" I know that I keep repeating myself about the canine connection and the pancreatic/IBS research connection, but just look at these FODMAPs and ask yourself if dogs eat these food items in their steady diets. Here are a few quick examples, but we will be more specific as we go along here. Does your dog readily eat onions (almost poisonous for dogs), avocados, cherries, peaches, garlic, almonds, apples, tomatoes, artichoke, cabbage, cauliflower, broccoli, grapes, pears, plumbs, blackberries, jams made from fruits, dried fruits, diet candies or diet chocolate (chocolate is dangerous for dogs), sugary sodas, sweet cakes, etc.?

At this current location along your digestive journey, you have already covered a lot of ground. There is no doubt that you encountered an awful lot of technical terminology and complex biochemical medical information during your journey. Clearly I am worried that you will either lose interest, become frustrated, or become overwhelmed by the material I have presented so far. As we look at and compare our parallel analogy to that of the automobile, we should take a look at your attitude toward your car.

There is no question that many Americans have love affairs with their cars. We are a mobile society, and aside from the necessity of a car for transportation, we also look at our automobiles as part of our family. We like our cars for aesthetics in addition to functionality. We want them to look pristine, clean, shiny, and in top shape. A majority of us take our cars in for regular scheduled service, keep them washed and waxed or put a protective sealer on the paint, and if a warning light appears on the dashboard digital display, we immediately take the car in for service. Ask yourself how complex the mechanics of your car are. How vigilant are you in keeping your car functioning optimally? Consider the financial aspects. How rare has it been for you not to perform a repair or service because of cost, even if it is necessary or indicated? More than likely, your credit card comes to the rescue. Do you make an effort to understand what the mechanic or service writer is saying?

Car owners are aware of the cooling system and coolant, fuel, oil, transmission fluid, windshield washer fluid, battery, brake fluid, etc. Consider whether you address your body in the same fashion and with the same concern. Your body is a functioning machine that deserves equal, if not greater, attention. Do you exercise a double standard between your car's well-being and that of your body?

Please do not assume that all physicians receive the same training—or should I say the same knowledge and experience—from their years in medical school, internship, and residency. I am not criticizing physicians or medicine at all. What I am saying is that not every human being possesses the same attributes and abilities. For this exact reason, some physicians are excellent diagnosticians, while others are mediocre. You could say the same goes for automobile mechanics or any other professional. We all excel in different areas, and it is your job as a patient to make an educated decision as to whether you are receiving optimal care or a correct diagnosis. If you do have IBS and are not attaining relief from or abatement of symptoms, then it is time to make a change.

If you were to look at Google Maps and see where you are now and where you have traveled, you could clearly see the complexities of the amazing machine we call the human body. Don't kid yourself; your car has its share of complexities too. So let's finish our journey and start to examine where the process can go wrong, how it can affect you, why it can cause IBS, and how to correct it.

To refresh your memory, you are in the duodenum and the chyme just arrived from the stomach. The chyme was ground, chopped up, bathed in gastric juices that contained hydrochloric acid, exposed to amylase to start the breakdown of starches, lipase to break down fats, and pepsin to break down proteins. This action was no different from mixing the batter you made in your mixing bowl for your cake that contained eggs, baking powder, cream of tartar, yeast, flour, chocolate chips, milk, vanilla, sugar, and coconut.

The chyme in the duodenum received a different bath. The pancreas delivered sodium bicarbonate, and the liver delivered bile into the duodenum in order to make a comfortable environment for the delivery of the pancreatic enzymes and intestinal enzymes. If the pH did not eventually rise to 8.0–8.5 and remained acidic, then the enzymes would be destroyed. Now for the added complexities. In addition to the nine enzymes that your pancreas delivered to the duodenum, the brush border cells on the villi tips dump additional enzymes into the duodenal mix of chyme.

Stop for a moment and look around where you are. You are in a mountainous region. The lining of the duodenum is not flat like the folds in the stomach. This region (i.e., the duodenum) is lined with microvilli. Located on the villi are some very specialized cells that are called brush border glandular cells. There are six major types of these; the previous chart showed the names of the enzymes they produce and their functions.

Now we are at the point in discussing what can and does go wrong, and why many physicians do not understand the situation because of past research and the way the results were taught in medical school.

CHAPTER 4

All of the Pieces Fit Together, Which Answers the IBS Question

Do you ever wonder why you develop a sore abdominal feeling or a burning sensation in your upper or lower GI tract? I am not talking about hyperacidity or a burning in your stomach. If you have IBS, you will know what I mean. If you don't have IBS, you still can imagine what I am talking about. Just think back to the last time you had a virus accompanied by diarrhea or vomiting. Think of how many times you had what you felt was food poisoning. After your infection is over and you start to recover, what does the lining of your intestines feel like? Do you feel like the intestinal lining is sensitive, sore, and raw? Do you get a burning feeling if you don't eat bland, mild food? Does it feel as if you can feel the food brush the walls of your intestines as it moves through your digestive tract? Just think about what it's like to suffer an abrasion on your arm from scraping your skin raw. Imagine putting alcohol on that raw skin to kill the bacteria that could cause an infection.

Why does this feeling occur? The answer is the holy grail to understanding IBS. This discussion requires you to look at the surface lining of the three sections of the small intestine: the duodenum, jejunum, and ilium. Your entire small intestine has a single-cell-thick lining that is topped with a protective mucus covering. When I started discussing the duodenum, the first section of your small intestine, I referred to it as the mountainous region because of its fingerlike projections, called villi. The tips of the villi contain the brush border cells of the single-cell layer of the mucosal lining of your small intestine. The cells that line the small intestines are called enterocytes, and they are truly unique. They go through a shedding or sloughing process every two to six days. This means that the lining of your intestine is normally constantly being replaced. Your exterior skin also is in a constant state of sloughing or shedding of the extreme outer surface of your skin. Your skin and the mucosal lining of your entire digestive tract have nerve endings that constantly communicate with your brain.

It is important to understand this process and the function of the villi lining your small intestine. Think about surface area. A flat surface has far less square footage than a surface covering the same area that has elevations, ridges, etc. This topography increases surface area. Nature created this feature to provide the maximum digestive and absorbent processing area in a small space. The villi increase the surface area for the body's digestive functions.

The gatekeeper is the lining of your small intestines—the single-cell layer of enterocytes topped with a mucus coating. I know that it is hard to believe, but your small intestine has a humongous bacterial population. In actuality there are ten times more microbes in the small intestine than the total number of cells in the human body. There are estimates that anywhere from five hundred to ten thousand species of bacteria live in our intestines. To complicate matters, friend and foe alike exist within this humongous bacterial population. The gatekeepers, your friends the enterocytes, prevent the bad guys (i.e. the pathogenic [disease causing] bacteria), from crossing the lining of the intestines and getting into other parts of the body. The mucus coating on the enterocyte lining is provided by the goblet cells, which are part of the array of the brush border cells that produce mucous. The second function of the enterocytes is to control osmotic pressure and permeability. What that means is that they control the ebb and flow of fluid in and out of the intestine.

Yes, this is complicated, but so is your car. Suppose you get into your car, turn the key, and hear *dat, dat, dat* and your engine does not turn over. You turn on the radio, and it works fine. Also the interior lights turn on. You think it can't be the battery because all of those things work. You decide to call a mechanic for assistance. Unfortunately, you can't get anyone, and you end up calling a local gas station that is not the most reputable. The mechanic comes out and says after looking under the hood, "Oh, it's your alternator." He replaces it and the battery and gives you a large bill. If you had been educated in this area or you thought to look at the date of your battery, you might have saved yourself a lot of money.

You were fooled by the radio and lights working, but the truth is that for that short duration, those things did not draw much electricity, whereas to start an engine requires a lot of amperage. If you saw the age of your battery or you remembered that it was five years old, you might have realized that it likely needed replacement. Being well educated in digestion is your first line of defense against IBS. Understanding disease, autoimmunity, and digestion will aid you in seeking a resolution to your condition of IBS. This book is mainly about IBS, but I should also mention inflammatory bowel disease (IBD). Inflammation is an integral consideration in studying and discussing disease.

In order to understand why you develop IBS and other gastrointestinal discomforts and disorders, you must understand disease and understand how medicine is structured and managed. Medicine is a very rigidly controlled profession that does not easily yield to change.

In medicine, when theories, new modalities, new treatments, and new approaches to disease and disorders come on the scene, acceptance will be a long and hard-fought battle toward acceptance, even if they prove to be viable.

It might become boring, intimidating, and repetitive to see the word "review" appear again, but it is essential to understand the process of digestion. Just as baking a complex cake requires diligence, adherence to a detailed recipe, and follow-through with the detailed directions, so must the rules of digestion be considered. From the moment your food enters the mouth until it reaches the end of the colon, it goes through coordinated, orchestrated, and detailed metabolic and digestive processes.

Now that you have spent time in the duodenum and have observed the digestive processes of breaking down chyme into its various smaller components and molecules, you can clearly see that nearly 60 percent of the digestive process occurs here. What failure actually can occur here, and how can that pose a problem for IBS?

This is the key to the etiology of IBS. To make it easy for you to understand, just read the overview below of the duodenum's comprehensive action.

1. The acidic chyme arrives in the duodenum.
2. The brush border cells provide secretin to stimulate the pancreas to introduce its necessary enzymes into the duodenum via the pancreatic duct.
3. The pancreas goes into action and dumps its enzymes through the pancreatic duct into the duodenum; the most important is sodium bicarbonate. The liver evacuates the gallbladder,

providing bile. These initial actions transform chyme into an alkaline medium from an acidic medium.

4. Now the chyme is ready for all of the needed pancreatic enzymes and brush border enzymes that will aid in breaking down the chyme contents into smaller molecules and smaller sugars.

Number four is the lightning rod for IBS. The foods you eat that contain sucrose, glucose, galactose, maltose, fructose, isomaltose, and lactose contain large sugar molecules that arrive in the duodenum basically intact.

If you think back to when we started to discuss how medicine arrived at its theory concerning pancreatitis and the possible connection to IBS, you can now understand why their theory was flawed. They were hung up on lipase and fat metabolism, but you can clearly see that metabolism and digestion are very broad. When you think about IBS, you truly have to take into account the enzymatic action of breaking down the complex sugar molecules. Item number four mentions that the brush border enzymes are the "lightning rod." Be very clear that I am not ignoring the enzyme amylase, which is produced in your saliva in addition to your pancreas. Amylase's main function is helping to break down starches.

Remember the comparison of the canine diet with the human diet? The human diet is broad and encompasses a wider variety of foods than that of the canine. Probably the easiest way to understand this concept is to create a meal example that would create an IBS-like response. Before we do that, we must assume and state that the patient has some degree of compromised brush border cells and or exocrine pancreatic cells that lost their ability to produce enough enzymes to break down the complex sugars into smaller molecules. As you look at the two meals below, think, "My dog doesn't eat these foods—certainly not in the quantity that the twenty-first-century American does"!

You must being thinking, "Why does this occur?" I will discuss this later, but it is now time to finish your digestive tour. Now for your meal. Let me provide an example of a lunch and dinner. Say you went to a Mexican restaurant and ate guacamole with onions, a cheese quesadilla with sour cream, onions, cheese, tomatoes, avocado, and refried beans. For dessert you went to a juice bar and had a smoothie consisting of blackberries, raspberries, peaches, and cherries with yogurt. For dinner you had a salad with onions, garlic, avocados, tomatoes, and beans with a creamy garlic dressing. The main course was fish sautéed in butter topped with a cheese cream sauce containing garlic and onions.

Now what happens? Those meals mentioned above arrive in the duodenum, but "Houston, we have a problem." We are lacking most of the brush border enzymes to start breaking down the large complex sugars in this food mix. Since these foods all escape the digestive process as a result of insufficient or nonexistent brush border chemicals—such as cholecystokinin, which stimulates digestion of proteins and fats; secretin, which controls secretions of the duodenum and osmoregulation; sucrase, which converts sucrose to disaccharides and monosaccharides; maltase, which converts maltose to glucose; lactase, which converts lactose to glucose and galactose; and, last, isomaltase, which converts maltose to isomaltose—what will happen here?

Of course you know the answer! Let the party begin. You just erected the duodenal brewery. You started the process of making your own signature brew. It starts here as you fire up the feeding frenzy for your resident bacteria. You are in essence brewing your ingested complex sugars, which are lacking exposure to the brush border enzymes that a normal person produces.

Guess what? You are just a little more than halfway through your digestive journey. Oh, look at your GPS. Get ready, because you are about to leave the duodenum and proceed into the jejunum. At this juncture, you would have normally experienced almost two-thirds of the digestion of your chyme and the broken-down essential nutrients that would have passed through your mucosa into your bloodstream and other systems for energy and other essential functions.

What happens at this stage if your FODMAPs are not exposed to the necessary enzymes while in the duodenum and leave the duodenum not broken down? Gas, cramping, bloating, and all of the other IBS symptoms will follow.

CHAPTER 5

What Is in Store for Us Now?

Having just arrived in the jejunum, the second section of the small intestine, you take a look around. It looks pretty much the same as the duodenum, except the microvilli are actually longer. What is most important to understand is that the rest of the majority of your digestion will be completed here. Absorption of the remaining nutrients, such as proteins, carbohydrates, amino acids, sugars, fatty acids, vitamins, electrolytes (salts), and water occurs here. They get transferred to the blood vessels that are attached to your duodenum and jejunum, where the nutrients are carried to your liver and then to the rest of your body.

Now remember that our friends and foes, the resident bacteria, are living here too. When you think about those guys, think about all of those large sugar molecules that are still present in the chyme and are not broken down if you present with IBS. Now your brewery, which was overworked in the duodenum, sets up shop in your jejunum because of the sugars not being broken down. It will continue the brewing of more of unwanted products (i.e., carbon dioxide, possibly hydrogen gas, and alcohol) that will add to the gas, cramps, and lose stools.

Take a look at the timeline of the food transiting past the stomach, small intestine, and large intestine. This will give you a good indication of how your food goes through the process of digestion and where the IBS patient encounters trouble and difficulty during the body's digestive process. I won't go into detail here, because I have already covered the details.

The Stomach
The food generally remains here for two to five hours for the production of chyme. Your stomach uses its muscles to churn and break up the food into smaller chunks or pieces along with adding digestive enzymes and exposing the food to acid. As chyme is produced, your stomach ejects small portions of chyme, about every twenty seconds, into the duodenum.

The Duodenum
From the time the chyme starts to arrive in the duodenum until it exits the ilium (last section of the small intestine) is a time span of approximately three to five hours. As the chyme arrives in the duodenum, the brush border cells release two hormones: secretin and cholecystokinin (CCK). These two hormones stimulate the pancreas to introduce sodium bicarbonate into the duodenum to neutralize the acidic chyme, and CCK also stimulates the liver to produce bile to help stabilize fat and aid in fat and vitamin absorption. During this period of time, the chyme is further broken down into smaller molecules and components, including the large sugars. As already discussed, the brush border cells produce and release their enzymes to complete digestion. The presence of the goblet cells produce and provide the mucus necessary to lubricate and protect the mucosal lining.

The Jejunum

This second section of the small intestines has a very large bacterial population, and the rest of the majority of digestion and the breakdown of those large sugar molecules continues. Now the pieces come together. In essence, ground zero for IBS is in the three sections of the small intestine. As the food which contains all of those complex sugars, moves from section to section of the small intestine, the breweries (bacterial colonies) come online if you can't produce the necessary brush border enzymes to break down the sugars. Your IBS literally gets worse as the chyme moves from the duodenum to the jejunum to the ilium. This occurs because the sugars remain intact, and as the bacterial population increases from duodenum to jejunum to ilium, so does the carbon dioxide and alcohol increase as the breweries work overtime, feeding on the sugars. The duodenum also contains a large amount of goblet cells, which produce mucus and help protect the chyme against acid. The major action of what I call microdigestion takes place here and in the ilium. What I mean is that the digestive action is occurring on a microscopic molecular level, meaning that this stage of digestion is the breaking down of large molecules of food components into smaller molecules. Examples are large sugars, such as sucrose, maltose, fructose, and lactose. Normally these large complex sugars are broken down by your body here if the brush border cells are functioning normally.

By the way, those who are lactose intolerant have their difficulties arise here and in the ilium, as they are unable to produce lactase. Lactase is an enzyme produced by a brush border cell that breaks down lactose, or milk sugar. The resultant sharp pain is due to the production of carbon dioxide and possibly hydrogen gas from lactobacillus bacteria working on the milk sugar (lactose) by digesting it (fermenting it), and that is why lactose intolerant people suffer.

The Ilium

Remember that the populations of bacteria become consistently larger
as you go from the duodenum to the jejunum to the ilium. What this
means is that your discomfort and symptoms worsen as you move
through the small intestine, because more and more bacteria are
feeding on the undigested sugars, in turn producing more gas. Peyer's
patch cells, a form of lymphoid tissue, is present in the ilium and is
responsible for providing leukocytes, a type of white blood cell that
fights infection. This last section of your small intestine is where a
majority of absorption of food nutrients and liquid takes place.

The Large Intestine

By the time the chyme is ready to leave the ilium, most of the nutrients
have been removed and absorbed into the blood supply that carries
them to the liver and then to the rest of the body. The remaining
substance is now basically waste and water. The main function of
the large intestine is reclamation of water for the body and removal
of salts. The large intestine holds over four hundred different species
of bacteria and quite possibly the highest concentration of bacteria in
any ecosystem. Of course, if you have IBS, then gas enters the large
intestine with the chyme. By the time the residue of the chyme reaches
the large intestine and carries with it some of the large sugars that
were not metabolized, it will provide a food source for the massive
amount of bacteria present.

You might wonder why I went into such detail concerning the
explanation of digestion. The answer is that those who suffer from
IBS are rarely given a plausible explanation of what IBS is or what
causes it. It still perplexes me that medicine has not addressed IBS in
this manner. Now that you have learned how your symptoms were
created, it is time to discuss why people develop IBS and how to
treat it.

CHAPTER 6

Why Do People Develop IBS?

I believe I have the answer, and my answer is based on several factors. Before I discuss how one develops IBS, it is necessary for you to understand the basic tenets of disease and understand the theories of pathogenesis (development of disease). It is far beyond my ability to establish an analogy in this case, such as the process of baking bread or the functioning of an automobile engine, because of the complexities of pathogenesis.

What is pathogenesis and why is it relevant in discussing IBS? Often when we human beings deal with something on a daily basis that is always present and always with us, we never give it a second thought. We approach living in a body in the same fashion and rarely give disease a second thought other than acceptance and hope that there is a cure. We often talk about the extreme complexities of the endless functions and systems of the human body, but the truth is that science does not have all the answers as of now. Nor has science attained all of the discoveries waiting to be made out there.

Human beings unfortunately understand the concept of war far too well. You might never give it a second thought, but your own body is constantly under siege and is fighting multiple major wars at the same time on a daily basis. There are two major front lines on the battlefield. The first is in and on the largest organ of your body—your skin. The skin, which is the outer covering of your body, is the first line of defense against pathogens that are always at your body's front door. They are awaiting entry into your body any way they can find an opening. An abrasion or scrape, a fissure, a tear, a clogged hair follicle, a pore on the skin containing excess oil or debris, or any other compromise to your skin can afford pathogens easy entry. It might be hard to believe, but quite often you come in contact with pathogens via physical contact, and they are usually present on your skin. If you think for a moment about how you are exposed to pathogens on a daily basis, you will realize how complex the action is of exposure to a pathogen developing into a full-blown infection.

How often do we stop to think about how our modern day lives expose us to pathogens? Most of us rarely do so. Believe it or not, the digital age offers several conduits for pathogens. Examples are use of computer keyboards that have multiple users at work, telephones in hotels and offices that have multiple users, electronic pens at credit card processing terminals, shopping carts in grocery stores, and magazines spread out in the waiting rooms in doctors' offices. Naturally our greatest defense is vigilant hand washing and conscious effort not to touch our faces. An easy access point for pathogens is your nose and its nasal passage.

Before we discuss the second front line battlefield, let us look at what "pathogenesis" means and what pathogens are. Pathogenesis is the production and development of disease, and a pathogen is a disease-causing agent, such as a virus, bacterium, or other microscopic organism. One last term you should know is "virulence." "Virulence" refers to the potential for a specific organism to cause disease and can signify its strength. This term is particularly important when discussing how aggressive a cancer is, how quickly a viral or bacterial infection develops, or literally how ill one becomes from an infection.

We often describe how virulent a specific type or species of bacteria or virus is known to be in causing infection. You might even hear on the news "Oh, this is a particularly virulent strain of the virus causing the flu this year." Examples of virulent pathogens are Ebola virus, HIV, yellow fever, mumps, and polio.

How virulence relates to IBS should be considered in trying to understand how we fight disease and the aftermath of the battle that we succumb to when the infection is over. I am referring here to resultant damage. I will give you some prime examples of this issue. A good example is heart damage that is sustained from a rheumatic fever infection. This infection is caused by the bacterium streptococcus, which leaves scarring in the heart valves as its aftermath. Naturally the heart valves function improperly after infection. Another example is measles, which is caused by a virus. A measles infection in a child can eventually cause deafness in the child.

Polio is caused by the poliomyelitis virus and can leave victims with permanent paralysis after fighting the virus. This example will help us discuss another aspect of disease. Aside from the degree of virulence, we must look at how we fight the pathogen.

Remember that your body is always under constant assault, and in normal situations, your body wins. In medicine we call a successful assault on the body an insult. A majority of the time, you never even realize that your body was engaged in a battle. If you were to truly monitor yourself, you would notice days when you did not feel up to par. When some people feel so, they may say, "I don't feel one hundred percent" or "I feel a little under the weather." Did you ever wonder why this occurs? For that matter, did you ever wonder why you develop a fever, joint pain, skin discomfort, achy eyes, headache, or any of the other numerous symptoms that we call feeling sick?

This occurs because of one of the numerous battles your body succumbs to when fighting off pathogens and even allergens. It can translate into a minor episode, akin to a local uprising that quickly gets squelched in a small country where people take up arms and try to depose a leader, or it can be like a major battle between countries, involving heavy armored tanks, heavy artillery, and aircraft dropping bombs. I won't discuss what the end possibilities are, as you have likely read them one thousand times. Of course you know what the various outcomes can be. Well, don't think for a second that your body does not parallel the same scenarios. Believe it or not, this is the key to understanding IBS.

One important factor to understand is the actual action your body takes in fighting a pathogenic infection. Only recently has medicine been investigating and trying to understand inflammation. When inflammation occurs in your body, it is a response to a pathogenic assault, insult from an injury to your body, or system failure. Inflammation is an action that is instituted and facilitated by your body's immune system. Just as countries manufacture bombs and war matériel, your body in essence does the same thing. Your body has in its arsenal various white blood cells, such as macrophages and lymphocytes. The macrophages, the so-called Pac-Man cells, attack, gobble up, and engulf pathogens—the viruses and bacteria that proliferate and attack the body's systems and or organs.

Under normal conditions, your immune system is active and present everywhere in your body, ready at a moment's notice to answer your body's beck and call. Unfortunately not everyone's immune system functions the same; some people's immune systems are compromised, and therefore their bodies do not launch as a good a fight as another person's. On the other hand, some immune systems overreact and attack more than just pathogens. They go on to attack the body itself; this is known as autoimmune disease. Now that it has been established that everyone is not created equal when it comes to immunity, we should look at some good examples and try to understand immunity a little better.

If you study what it was like during the polio epidemics before the early 1950s and the aftermath of those who succumbed to polio infection, you will realize that there were varying degrees of severity and also varying degrees of sustained damage among polio victims. Why was it that some people recovered from the polio infection and did not sustain any damage or aftereffects, while others would never walk again, and others ended up not being able to breathe on their own, forced to remain on respirators? The answer lies in their immune systems.

You might also wonder why some people rarely become ill while others keep succumbing to illnesses. You might also wonder why some people sustain infections and recover much quicker than the average person. It all has to do with how well the person's onboard army (i.e., immune system) is armed and mobilized. Trying to understand disease is truly the last frontier because it entails understanding genetics, the immune system, inflammation, DNA, polymorphism, and many other factors. Rest assured that I will not delve deeply into these influences on disease. My goal here is to explain what happens and how it relates to the cause of IBS.

To make it easy for you to understand the action and progression of disease, I should explain how vaccines prevent disease. In disease there are two distinct armies: the antigens (the bacteria, viruses, and other micro-organisms that cause disease) and the antibodies (the agents your immune system creates in response to the pathogens in order to kill them).

An example is the polio vaccine. Here is how it works. Since the poliomyelitis virus is very virulent, many people have difficulty developing an antibody to fight and kill the virus. Hence they end up suffering paralysis, as the poliomyelitis virus destroys the motor neurons. Medicine developed a vaccine against the virus by creating an attenuated vaccine. This means they altered, weakened, and made the virus less virulent. The virus they were left with was basically intact but incapable of reproducing or replicating itself; nor could it cause disease. In simple language, it stimulates your body's immune system to produce specific poliomyelitis virus antibodies that your immune system specifically designs against the poliomyelitis virus that remains in your body. These antibodies in essence remember the poliomyelitis virus, can recognize any future potential poliomyelitis virus intruder, and now know how to destroy it before it can replicate itself and cause the disease. This vaccination provides you with protection against any future polio viral attack.

In normal daily living, your body performs this action on its own. Again, remember that everyone's immune system is not identical. Immune functionality varies just like hair color, eye color, height, and skin color. This variability is caused by genetics, and genetics plus immune history plays a much larger role in disease then we realize. By now you are aware that IBS is governed by genetic influences that impact the body's ability to fight disease. However, it goes much further then you likely realize. What I am talking about is autoimmune response disease.

CHAPTER 7

The Role of Autoimmune Response Disease in IBS

You will now find all the answers to your questions. Let me be very clear concerning IBS. The condition is quite different from that of the average disease a person can contract, and to make matters worse, it presents with multiple symptoms and varies in intensity and duration. Also, there could feasibly be more than one cause—theoretically up to twenty-six causes. The reason for this is, as you now know, that there are at least twenty-six different digestive enzymes that are actively involved in the body's digestive processes. This means that if an immune response to a virus or bacterium in one of the four regions that produce digestive enzymes does not stop after winning the localized battle against a virus or bacterium and by accident goes on to destroy cells that are responsible for digestive enzyme production, then that is an autoimmune response and can contribute to IBS. This, of course, is theory and has not been proven by medical research.

Here I am referring to exocrine pancreatic enzyme insufficiency (EPEI) and intestinal enzyme insufficiency (IEI). I wish I could just provide you with easy explanations and answers, but life does have an awful lot of complexities, and they do not always have simple solutions.

To go further, I must define and discuss autoimmune disease. Autoimmune disease occurs when your body is exposed to a pathogen or illness and your body's immune system not only attacks that pathogen but also goes on to attack the body itself. There are several autoimmune diseases, and some are one-time events that just leave secondary damage—that is, damage to your body from your own body's immune system. Your immune system malfunctions and wrongly recognizes certain cells in your body as foreign antigens and destroys them.

An example of an autoimmune response disease is type 1 diabetes. Remember that genetics plays a major role in disease and it is indeed the case with Type 1 diabetes. People who develop Type 1 diabetes are genetically predisposed to the disease. This means that the person inherited a gene that, if activated, can induce the immune system to destroy the beta cells in the endocrine pancreas—the cells that produce insulin. This usually occurs after a major infection that requires a strong effort by your immune system to fight a pathogenic response. An example might be a severe streptococcus infection that lasts days with elevated temperatures, sore throat, gastrointestinal discomfort, chills, etc. If the streptococcus pathogen is very virulent, your immune system will most likely have to mount a major offensive to combat and beat the infection. Viruses can instigate similar responses.

So what happens that causes your immune system to go astray and start attacking your pancreas? Every cell in your body has certain markers on it. Without going into detail, they are akin to directional lights or switches in that they can act as gatekeepers and keep certain substances from crossing the cell wall while allowing others in. In terms of your immune system, you have lymphocytes, which are a variety of white blood cells traveling throughout your body in the bloodstream, lymph system, and what we call the interstitial fluid—the fluid that your cells and organs are bathed in. The theory is that after your immune system completes its aggressive fight to destroy the pathogens or antigens that caused an infection, it makes a mortal error and recognizes specific cell markers as foreign antigens instead of normal cells and attacks them. That is why a person who inherits the gene for potential diabetes is predisposed to developing diabetes. That person's immune system may become overzealous after fighting a streptococcus infection and attack the beta cells in the pancreas. The eventual destruction that occurs over several weeks to a few months renders the person permanently a type 1 diabetic. He or she will never again be able to regenerate those beta cells or produce insulin.

There are many other examples, such as rheumatoid arthritis, systemic lupus, multiple sclerosis, celiac disease, pernicious anemia, psoriasis, Addison's disease, and many others.

Why do I believe that autoimmune disease plays a role in IBS? It is assumed that IBD (Inflammatory Bowel Disease) is an autoimmune disease, so why wouldn't IBS follow suit? There have been recent studies and discoveries that support my theory. First I will give you my background, and then I will discuss the studies that prove my theory.

I have been a type 1 diabetic for forty-seven years. For the past twenty-nine years, I have been on an insulin infusion pump for the treatment of my type 1 diabetes. It is well known that diabetes is a disease and condition that causes major complications and damage to a diabetic's body. It is a chief cause of blindness, renal failure (kidney failure), neuropathy, amputations, and a host of other complications. These conditions arise out of poor control of the diabetic's blood sugar level.

Owing to my knowledge and diligent control of my blood sugar, I was able to avoid all of those complications.

In the year 2000, I was diagnosed with a large and virulent melanoma that was excised out of my arm, and I followed up with a type of chemotherapy that stimulated my immune system for one year and six months. I had to inject myself with GM-CSF. That stands for granulate macrophage-colony stimulating factor. Because melanoma does not respond to chemotherapy or radiation treatment, researchers theorized that if we could heighten the immune system to produce an excessive amount of macrophages (a type of white blood cell), then maybe the heightened aggressive immune system would seek out and destroy any renegade melanoma cell or cells that broke away from the tumor. This therapy stimulated the bone marrow to produce an excessive amount of macrophages.

I injected myself every day for two weeks on and two weeks off for eighteen months. With my immune system heightened, I ran low-grade fevers; suffered chills, lethargy, and gastrointestinal discomfort; and lost weight. My weight went down to 129 pounds, and my average weight had always been 145 pounds. After the therapy was over, the following year I contracted pancreatitis. I could theorize that the cause of the pancreatitis was from my immune system having been altered or influenced by the GM-CSF but, I will never know.

This is where it gets interesting. I eventually did recover and did have extensive testing done. At the time, my exocrine pancreas (the majority of the pancreas that produces digestive enzymes) was compromised. I had difficulty metabolizing fats and other foods. I lost weight and always felt ill owing to gastrointestinal difficulties. The symptoms eventually became intermittent, but I never recovered 100 percent. As time went on, I started to have more gastrointestinal difficulties and became intolerant of many more foods. My endocrinologist was insistent that I had celiac disease. I had negative test results for IgA and IgD, blood markers for celiac disease. I displayed symptoms of IBS, and I was referred to a gastroenterologist, and he performed a colonoscopy. His observations concluded that I did not have celiac disease. He said my intestinal villi were not blunted or flattened, which usually denotes celiac disease. His diagnosis was malabsorption and IBS. His form of treatment was probiotics.

As time went on, my symptoms became progressively worse. I started to believe that I was lactose intolerant and gluten intolerant. The IBS became more pronounced, and my diet became more restrictive. During this past decade, my endocrinologist who was treating me for my type1 diabetes told me that I probably have small intestinal bacterial overgrowth (SIBO). He said it was common in diabetics but the reason for this was unknown. Treatment was a round of special antibiotics named, Xifaxan.

One and a half years ago was the turning point. I was being treated by a new gastroenterologist, and he tested me for lactose intolerance. My test results were off the chart, but I still did not attain relief, so I decided to do my own extensive research. My gastroenterologist also diagnosed me with SIBO and treated me with Xifaxan. Since I had studied medicine my whole life and understood it, even though I never attended medical school or worked as a medical professional, I told myself that I could figure this out on my own.

I started doing research by adhering to an extremely restrictive diet and keeping an accurate diary of everything I ingested along with logging notes of my GI condition and my symptoms. I started to learn which foods were the offenders. Later I started a FODMAP diet, which in all honesty is extremely rigorous, restrictive, and difficult to maintain.

After one year's research in reading and studying medical journals, published research papers, medical abstracts, and presentations at international conventions on gastroenterology, I figured it out. After discussing all of this with my dear friend Steve Best, MD, who is a neuroscientist, researcher, and neuropsychiatrist, I received a positive opinion of my theory. He suggested that I read veterinary medical papers that had been published on pancreatitis. He felt that since science and medicine utilize the animal model extensively for medical studies, and particularly since veterinarians treat pancreatitis frequently, I could get good insight and develop a correlation between exocrine pancreatic enzyme insufficiency and IBS. When I did that, it became clear as day when I saw the correlation between pancreatitis and IBS.

This is where it became complicated and difficult to prove to many of my friends who are physicians in varied specialties of medicine. But in the early spring of 2015, I came across recently published medical papers that had been presented at the world endocrinology conferences in September 2014. These papers addressed new theories concerning the correlation between pancreatitis and diabetes. The evidence and concrete theories were so strong that the researchers classified a new disease—type 3c diabetes. This condition's symptoms present with pancreatic enzyme insufficiency as a primary symptom and the development of a secondary symptom of diabetes.

If we just institute deductive reasoning, we can easily deduce that it can't be assumed that the development of diabetes always presents as a secondary symptom of type 3c diabetes. Does the old saying "What came first, the chicken or the egg?" apply here? We must truly think outside the box in this case. It will require you to stop and look at disease with twenty-first-century thinking. You must ask yourself what is really going on in our lives, our society, and the world today in terms of disease and understanding disease.

Thomas A. Sessa, DVM, my dear friend who is a veterinarian and whom I spend Tuesdays with in the OR observing surgery, totally concurs with my theories and understands my correlation to how medicine reached its approach to digestive disorders.

Unless you never read newspapers, watch television, surf the Internet, or observe people in public, you must realize that we are going through a major shift in America in terms of an evolving health crisis. You hear the words, phrases, and terms every day: "childhood obesity," "type 2 diabetes," "metabolic syndrome," "morbid obesity," "gluten intolerance," "lactose intolerance," and "prediabetic children." Fifty years ago these modern terms were barely even conceived of. This is a major problem in America today, but since this book is about IBS, we will not delve into those topics here.

I will guarantee you that if you ask your general practitioner, endocrinologist, or gastroenterologist about type 3c diabetes, he or she will not have a clue about it. In getting back to my theory on the development of IBS, I must clearly address autoimmune response diseases.

You will recall the earlier discussion of the presence of natural living colonies of bacteria. You also should realize that there are friendly bacteria that are resident inhabitants along with the foes that are pathogenic bacteria. The mucosa lining the small and large intestines is composed of enterocytes, and the mucosal lining is epithelial tissue. The reason I bring this up is that the skin is also composed of epithelial cells. These linings are a first line of defense against pathogens that are at bay, waiting to attack the body. As I previously said, multiple wars and skirmishes are occurring on a daily basis in and around your body. Most of the time, you are not aware of these battles.

When the tides turn in favor of the pathogens and they get a foothold, an infection ensues. The pathogens are always opportunists and will always seize an entry point into your body to set up residence. It is up to your police force (your immune system) to keep them in check. As we all know, not every police force is created equal. Some have more available capital, some have better training, and some have better equipment available to combat crime. In essence, your body's immune system is no different. For this simple reason, some people rarely contract colds, stomach viruses, or flu, or even suffer from allergies, while others repeatedly succumb to illness. This is obviously due to how well one's immune system functions.

It is utterly absurd, in my view, to hold the notion that IBS is not a result of an autoimmune issue. If you take into account my particular case history, you should realize that I am not representative of the average IBS sufferer. Even though my case is unusual, the basic premise still applies. The action of the GM-CSF that heightened my immune system was an extreme situation, but what you must realize is that I was *predisposed* for an autoimmune reaction. I could include many published medical papers here to support my theory and what I am discussing now. When your body sustains an injury or an attack by an antigen, it usually responds with inflammation. The fact that I developed type 1 diabetes forty-seven years ago because I sustained a major streptococcus infection that resulted in an autoimmune response is, in my view, enough evidence that autoimmunity plays a role in IBS.

Let us take a look at what happens to a person who has IBS. First of all, did you ever wonder why "irritable" is part of the name? Usually when you have an irritable condition, it is not constant; "irritable" denotes that you have a sensitivity. A person who presents with IBS is usually on a roller coaster; by that I mean he or she goes through periods lasting from a week to ten days of discomfort accompanied by soft stool or diarrhea, frequent bowel movements, gas, bloating, a raw feeling in the lining of the intestine, and maybe even a burning feeling. Why does this occur? The simple answer is that the person's body reacts to one or more offending foods that have been ingested. More than likely, it was a food on the list of FODMAPs. How do these foods cause an insult to the body?

The insult is not directly caused by the food but is rather the result of the food. The simple fact is that the IBS patient's brush border cells have been compromised by an autoimmune reaction that occurred during one or more bouts with an antigen (i.e., a bacterium or virus within the small intestines, the exocrine pancreas, or both). If the patient's immune system has any degree of an autoimmune tendency, then it would be safe to assume that some of the patient's brush border cells were permanently destroyed or reduced in number by the patient's own antibodies. Remember: that can also apply to the patient's exocrine pancreas cells that produce digestive enzymes.

So how does this produce an IBS symptomatic reaction? It is the ingestion of those foods that contain high levels of FODMAPs—those complex sugars that start the process. Now for the complication: Remember that the enterocytes, those cells that line the small intestine, are shed every three to five days. If you have an excess of complex sugars present in your small intestine owing to intestinal enzyme insufficiency, you will experience a large blossom of bacteria overgrowth, and then a battle will occur in your small intestine to try to control the bacteria. If these bacteria become out of control and hamper the enterocytes from replenishing the mucosal lining, then you end up feeling pain, rawness, and soreness. Add to that the fact that you don't have the brush border enzymes to break down the complex sugars, so these overabundant bacteria act as a brewery. They start fermenting the complex sugars. This becomes an endless cycle of periods of calm followed by insults to the mucosa that result in temporary damage until the enterocytes replenish and the mucosa starts to furnish mucus to bathe, lubricate, and protect the intestine. This is why an IBS patient can achieve temporary remission if he or she adheres to an incredibly bland, strict diet that lacks any offending FODMAPs.

If you look at all of the digestive enzymes produced in the stomach, exocrine pancreas, and small intestine, you can clearly see that it is pure guesswork to try to ascertain where the digestive system is failing in the patient. To the best of my knowledge, diagnostic testing to determine which stomach cells, exocrine pancreatic cells, or brush border cells have been destroyed or compromised by an autoimmune response does not currently exist. For this exact reason, medicine still concentrates on chronic pancreatitis, which is currently diagnosed via testing, primarily looking for lipase insufficiency. The fecal tests done also look for unbroken down fat content. Sometimes they also measure amylase, which breaks down starches; but mainly medicine concentrates on fat absorption failure.

Hello! What about the other stomach, exocrine pancreatic, and intestinal enzymes? I have never seen this addressed in print!

Now that I have clearly stated my basic theory, I should explain a few more observations that can offer more support to my theory. Take a look at lactose intolerance. We all are very aware of this condition; we see it discussed all the time in the movies, television, print media, and advertising. Ever wonder why few know why people develop this condition? Of course you already know the answer, because you just read about the brush border cells and particularly the ilium (last section of your small intestine), where major lactose breakdown occurs.

The reason some become lactose intolerant is because the brush border cells that produce lactase (the enzyme that breaks down lactose, or milk sugar) no longer exist or are grossly impaired. Why would this happen? It would be safe to assume that cellular destruction or impairment is due to genetic involvement. One theory is that lactose intolerance is a normal progression of human development. Science theorizes that lactation is a natural function of human propagation and is in place after pregnancy to provide sustenance for the growth and development of the newborn until he or she is weaned off of mother's milk. The theory is that cow's milk is for baby cows. Yet we eat cheese, drink milk, and eat ice cream along with other dairy, so why does most of our population escape lactose intolerance? Think about this: certain groups of people, such as Asians and African Americans, are genetically predisposed to lactose intolerance. How many children, including African Americans, are not wild about milk or ice cream? How many children complain about stomachaches after consuming cheese, ice cream, or milk? Often they are aware of this connection and just unconsciously avoid dairy.

Now go one step further and ask yourself why some people are moderately lactose intolerant while others experience full-blown intolerance? Of course the answer is that it all depends on how many brush border cells are left to produce lactase. Yes, the ability to produce lactase equates to the degree of lactose intolerance.

In my view, it has to be directly correlated to genetics—and more specifically, genetic predisposition. I will go further and say that it is an autoimmune response reaction that dictates the degree of destruction of the specific brush border cells. The action of destruction could very well be connected to an immune reaction to a virulent lactobacillus infection. This scenario is most logical, and many physicians see temporary lactose intolerance in patients that have had very bad gastrointestinal infections. After several months after infection, most patients return to normal.

In the final section of this book, I will discuss treatment protocol. Considering how far medicine has advanced, it is entirely incomprehensible that medicine did not pursue this logical approach to understanding and treating IBS and SIBO (Small Intestinal Bacterial Overgrowth). I will clearly tell you that it took considerable time, deductive reasoning, and repetitive experimentation to develop my hypothesis for the etiology of IBS and its successful treatment protocol.

CHAPTER 8

An Effective Treatment Protocol for IBS

It is clearly obvious that you could possibly be suffering from exocrine pancreatic / intestinal enzyme insufficiency. Therefore, I propose to redefine and reclassify IBS by changing this disorder's label to EPIEI (Exocrine Pancreatic Intestinal Enzyme Insufficiency). This treatment protocol discussion will be divided into three specific areas:

1. personalized self-diagnosis, which includes an analysis of dietary intake;
2. titration of enzyme-replacement therapy (ERT) (i.e., the process of figuring out the proper dosage of ERT); and
3. the method and procedure of dispensing the ERT.

Again, I want to reiterate that I am not a physician; I am not diagnosing you or prescribing medication. What I am doing is presenting to you a compilation of research that I have done on my own from medical portals, published medical research, medical abstracts, medical papers, and, most important, myself-analysis and experimentation on myself. Medicine is unique in that it is not as exact a science as one might perceive, because the human being presents many variables. Just think about that! We are not exact carbon copies of each other. Take, for instance, a patient who presents with symptoms of hypothyroidism. This condition occurs when the thyroid gland is not producing enough of the hormone thyroxin. Does a physician automatically prescribe and dispense the exact same amount of the hormone replacement medication to every patient with this condition? Of course not. Each patient's deficient thyroid gland produces a different amount of thyroxin, and so the physician must titrate the dosage by starting off with a basic amount of micrograms of supplement and periodically run a blood test to guide the physician to increase the dosage until the patient achieves adequate thyroid activity.

You might wonder why medicine can't be exact and why dosages of medicine are not all the same for each given medical condition or patient. When a physician prescribes a prescription drug, he or she must also take into account the weight of the patient and prescribe the amount of medicine accordingly. A 189-pound patient certainly requires a greater amount of medication than a 90-pound patient. The medical treatment of human beings must utilize a variable method and approach to a specific condition. As I said, we are not all carbon copies of each other, and specific medical conditions do not present equally in the same fashion in each patient.

There are always varying degrees of intensity and symptoms that a physician must take into account before treating and prescribing medicine. An easy way to understand this is to remember the degrees of severity of polio damage, kidney infections, stomach viruses, etc. Each infection does not present with the same intensity or same virulence; nor does it cause the same insult or damage to the body.

I will address treatment for EPIEI in the same fashion. This approach and principle is based on how varied the symptoms of EPIEI or IBS are from patient to patient. It will be important for you to have a partnership or working relationship with your physician. As the patient, you cannot assume or self-diagnose, and therefore I prevail upon you to make sure that you are worked up via a physical examination and that the necessary blood work and other diagnostics are performed. I assume that those people who suffer from EPIEI have received a diagnosis of IBS from a physician and chose to read this book because they have not attained any abatement of symptoms or relief from their IBS.

Now let us begin on the road to accomplishing a marked improvement in your health and well-being. The first phase of this process will start with you becoming attuned to your body, which includes becoming observant of all foods that you eat and documenting all food intake and exhibited symptoms. This is the most important step in diagnosing and understanding why you develop or exhibit EPIEI. I will not fool you or mislead you concerning figuring out the cause of your EPIEI. It is a difficult and arduous task.

In order to perform this function, you must first institute a dietary change to facilitate the repair of the mucosal lining of your small and large intestines. I have covered this extensively in this book; this is what occurs to the lining of your small and large intestines after an insult to the enterocytes that make up your mucosal lining by the ingestion of offending foods. You must facilitate the repair process to your mucosal lining before you can start the process of deductive reasoning to determine your specific EPIEI. In essence you are striving to discover which digestive enzymes are deficient in your body.

Why do people feel they are riding a roller coaster when it comes to their digestive tracts? This is what is perplexing and drives patients crazy. They say, "Why can I go a week without any symptoms and then all of a sudden I feel sick and it lasts a week to ten days?" Some patients who have suffered from the condition for a long while take longer periods of time to recover between episodes. What adds to patients' frustration is that, in most instances, their physicians cannot offer a plausible answer.

But I do know the answer! The answer is connected to stability and fragility. I use those two words in reference to your single-cell intestinal lining. Just think about it. These enterocytes, that single-cell layer lining your small intestine, is sloughing cells all of the time and offering new replacements every two to five days. What do you think happens when there is an explosive bacterial overgrowth phenomenon? Those resident bacteria are not always friendly. If some of your brush border cells sustained damage from a pathogen or were permanently damaged from a major infection—such as severe gastroenteritis from E. coli, salmonella, or other bacterial infections—then you in all likelihood could become deficient in one or more intestinal enzymes.

Just think what happens to your arm after you sustain a bad scrape or abrasion and you keep damaging that same wound over and over. You repeatedly reopen the wound, lose the formed scab, bleed from the wound, and wait for your body to attempt repair and restore your skin again. Your intestinal mucosal lining goes through the same process.

If you have EPIEI, you know what I mean about the soreness you feel every time food passes through your intestine. The pain from the accompanying gas, cramps, and bloating of course comes from the fermentation of the complex sugars that failed to digest because of a lack of enzymes. How does the healing process start? A patient who has IBS or EPIEI unconsciously facilitates healing by losing the desire to eat or choosing a very bland diet because other food is a turnoff. This process unconsciously allows your macrophages and leucocytes, your white blood cells, to fight the pathogens. Inflammation occurs as a result of the presence of an infection and a compromised intestinal lining due to the body's immune fighting action. During the following ten days to two weeks, your intestinal lining goes through a healing process by trying to repair the damage through enterocyte cell replacement. If this cell layer sustains damage from bacteria or a viral infection, then spaces between the cells can allow gaps, providing openings for fluid and material exchange between the small intestine and the surrounding tissues. This, of course, can facilitate increased potential for the development of diarrhea.

The brush border cells can be replenished too. Just think how you feel after fighting a stomach virus. After the first day of recovery, do you want to dive into a buffet or Sunday brunch? I highly doubt that!

Step I

Your initial task is to purchase a calendar or diary that has lined pages and lists dates. It must be large enough to allow you to log all of the foods, snacks, and drinks that you consume each day, along with the times at which you consume them. That means each meal, each snack, and each drink must be logged. During this process, I want you to avoid all FODMAPs. These are foods that contain large, complex sugar molecules (e.g., onions, avocados, garlic, cherries, peaches, cauliflower, broccoli, apples, blackberries, grapes, fruit juices, plums, pears, dried fruits, nectarines, watermelon, asparagus, artichokes, cabbage, beans, garlic, diet drinks, diet candy, and artificial sweeteners). You must be very careful with any salad dressings and sauces. Please read labels, as many foods have hidden added ingredients. You must avoid any so-called Tex-Mex food served in your favorite Mexican-style restaurants and avoid dining out, where you cannot determine any potentially unwanted hidden ingredients in the meal.

Please remember that this is the test phase for enzyme deficiencies only.

This is not an easy task. Believe me; I know. You must do this for a minimum of two full weeks—preferably one month. During this time you must log *all* of your bathroom functions, including the consistency of all of your stools and frequency of bowel movements. Also list any symptoms of gas, cramping, bloating, sharp pain, or soreness or tenderness in your intestinal lining. Step I is a very important task and diagnostic tool. Unfortunately medicine currently does not have another viable option to make a diagnosis that would be easier on you. This procedure does not have a set time span for attaining a diagnosis, because the degree of severity is contingent on several factors: the degree of severity of damage to your mucosal lining, which includes the length of time the lining of your small intestine was in crisis; which cells were compromised or destroyed (i.e., brush border cells or enterocytes); and, finally, when you last exhibited normal digestive functionality.

The successful results of this diagnostic testing protocol are contingent upon your participation and willingness to strictly follow the restrictive requirements of the test. I am sure it will not be too hard for you to figure out if you are lactose intolerant, but I suggest that you refrain from eating any dairy unless it is lactose free during this phase. You must approach the diagnostic phase with deductive reasoning. This also means you may not ingest butter or foods fried in butter. You may have no cream sauces or desserts made with dairy. In essence you are practicing an elimination diet. This will accomplish two things. First, you are facilitating the healing of the mucosal lining of your small intestine by eliminating potential foods that can cause insults and injury to your intestinal lining. In addition, you are possibly reducing the bacterial population by cutting off their excessive food supply—those large, complex sugar molecules—which will prevent the fermentation process. The second function is that you are preparing your body for Step II. This will be the reintroduction of specific food types back into your digestive system.

We are still discussing the initial diagnostic phase. Once your body has become devoid of the offending foods that cause bodily insults and your intestinal lining achieves total healing, then you can proceed to Step II. But here is one very important consideration: starting Step II purely depends upon the degree of damage that your intestinal lining has sustained. Gluten intolerance can play a role here too. I chose to eliminate gluten from my diet because my endocrinologist was so insistent in his belief that I had celiac disease. There is a high propensity for diabetics to develop celiac disease or become gluten intolerant. This Step I test scenario might appear to be draconian, but unfortunately current medicine has not developed useful diagnostics to test for the presence or absence of maltase, sucrase, isomaltase, lactase, and many other enzymes. Therefore, Step II uses the reintroduction of one specific food component at a time to see if it will elicit a noticeable response.

I am sure that the mention of gluten draws attention. Please rest assured that this is a commentary on the American diet. There have been a lot of accusatory comments and opinions in the medical community and in the media concerning the efficacy of gluten intolerance. Since I have been gluten free for one year, I will briefly explain my observations and feelings from this past year as well as the benefits I have received from the avoidance of gluten. In addition, I will explain in a separate chapter the quandary that gluten presents to the American public and how the gluten issue arose.

Now let's return to your quest to rid yourself of pain, suffering, and discomfort. If you were to look back in your mind and superficially review the material you have read to date, you can clearly see that your digestive system is in a constant state of flux and always under siege. As you begin this elimination diet test, you are confronting the previous description head on.

Of course I know the first question that is on the tip of your tongue: "How long will this test take?" The answer entails how long have you *consistently* and *continuously* experienced your symptoms without a hiatus or holiday. After experiencing an episode, how long does it take you to feel normal again? One important issue is whether you currently have or ever had an autoimmune response disease, allergies, or persistent infections. If so, how quickly did you or do you recover from any of these?

We must be vigilant and strong in carrying this test through to a clear and symptom-free homeostasis in order to begin the diagnostic process. An extreme example is in those who recently discover that they have celiac disease. This is an inherited disease; a person is genetically predisposed to developing the disorder. The patient becomes unable to digest and metabolize wheat protein, and his or her immune system actually attacks his gastrointestinal tract. One of the telltale diagnostic symptoms is that the small intestinal villi become blunted and flattened from the autoimmunological response to the gluten. I mention this because after the patient goes on a gluten-free diet, it can easily take up to one year or more for his or her mucosal lining to return to normal—if it can. Celiac patients can even become malnourished from the damage to the villi and the brush border cells. Their food absorption can become grossly impaired and compromised because of the damage done to the villi.

As you can see, discussing EPIEI is not an exact science, owing to the amount of variables that are encountered. This consideration makes treatment so difficult for the attending physician and the patient. How do you measure what damage has been sustained by the mucosa after an episode or outbreak caused by a reaction to an offending food? How does the physician ascertain where the damage occurred and what exocrine pancreatic or brush border cells were compromised or damaged? The truth is that there is no reliable test that is available to the physician. Naturally an endoscopy can be performed, and the villi can be observed. If the gastroenterologist does not observe flattened or blunted villi, then he or she assumes that the patient does not have celiac disease. Of course a blood test for the markers IgA and IgD would offer confirmation too. Unfortunately, to the best of my knowledge, a biopsy is not performed to observe the villi on a microscopic cellular level in order to view the brush border glandular cells or lack thereof.

Endoscopy can reach the first section of the small intestine, the duodenum, to determine whether the brush border is compromised, but it can do so only visually—not on a cellular microscopic level. Now with the advent of ingestible pill cameras, viewing the brush border mucosal lining of the duodenum, jejunum, and ilium can be possible. There are risks with the possibility of the pill cam lodging itself in a pocket or fold of the small intestine, in turn causing an obstruction. For those who suffer with diverticulosis or diverticulitis, the use of the pill cam can offer increased risk.

Setting Up My Diagnostic Log

Here is an example of what you should strive for in creating your diagnostic log.

Thursday July 29, 2015

Notes: Today is day one of my elimination diet.

7:00 a.m. I feel bloated, have sharp pain and cramping, and my intestinal lining feels sore. My stool was lose, smelly, and gaseous. After evacuation, my colon felt very sore.

7:30 a.m. Breakfast:
1/4 cup cantaloupe, two poached eggs, two slices of gluten-free bread, two cups of coffee with one packet of sugar each (no artificial sweetener)

10:30 a.m. Bathroom visit. Same symptoms as at 7:00 a.m.

12:30 p.m. Lunch:
One tuna fish sandwich on gluten-free bread with lettuce and mayonnaise, one iced tea (no artificial sweetener)

2:30 p.m. Bathroom visit. Same reoccurring symptoms. Have felt gassy all day.

3:30 p.m. Ate a peanut butter cracker snack brought from home.

5:00 p.m. Bathroom visit. Felt more cramping, gas, and small, projectile, soft stool.

5:00–6:00 p.m. Felt rawness and soreness in my intestinal tract.

7:00 p.m. Dinner:
salad (green lettuce with olive oil and vinegar, a few walnuts, and a few strawberries), a baked potato with margarine, grilled chicken with olive oil and herbs, oil, zucchini

8:45 p.m. Felt less cramping and distention, but still felt urgency. Bathroom visit. Smaller loose messy stool not formed. Same sore, raw feeling.

11:00 p.m. Had lemon ices before bed.

Friday July 30, 2015

6:50 a.m. My current condition is much the same as yesterday, except the cramping is markedly reduced. I was still gassy but not as intensely as yesterday. Stool was soft and not formed.

7:15 a.m. Breakfast:
half a cup of strawberries, scrambled eggs cooked in margarine, coffee with sugar

11:00 a.m. Bathroom visit. Soft stool and minimal gas. I still felt that my intestinal lining was sore.

12:15 p.m. Lunch:
hamburger without a bun, rice crackers with margarine from home, iced tea

3:55 p.m. Snack:
lactose-free cheese

4:15 p.m. Bathroom visit. Soft stool, minimal gas. Soreness was less, but awareness still present.

6:35 p.m. Dinner:
baked salmon with olive oil, herbs, and lemon slices; quinoa; salad (shredded carrots, lettuce, and cherry tomatoes with oil and vinegar)

9:30 p.m. Snack: gluten-free pretzels

10:00 p.m. Bathroom visit. Very minimal gas, and stool was small and not as soft.

Saturday July 31, 2015

7:00 a.m. I awakened without soreness. I did not have a sense of urgency to use the bathroom.

7:30 a.m. Breakfast:
oatmeal with margarine, coffee with lactose-free milk and sugar, dish of raspberries

8:00 a.m. Bathroom visit. Felt better—no gas or cramping, and stool was smaller and less voluminous.

12:30 p.m. Lunch:

lactose-free cheese, banana, mixed nuts (no almonds)

6:20 p.m. Dinner:

steak with rice and spinach, mixed greens salad

7:30 p.m. Bathroom visit. Noticeable difference. No discomfort and very small stool, formed but not firm.

I think you are able to understand the concept and intent here. This task of performing an elimination diet is the key to facilitating the healing process of your mucosa (i.e., the intestinal lining). As discussed previously, the intent is to discover which exocrine pancreatic or intestinal brush border cell enzymes are deficient in your body. As per the above format, you must carry on keeping this log until *all* of your symptoms have abated and disappeared. When your stool formation returns to normal, you no longer experience that sore feeling in your intestinal lining, and you no longer produce gas, then you know that the healing process has been reasonably advanced.

It is my contention that EPEI (Exocrine Pancreatic Enzyme Insufficiency) plays a lessor role in so-called IBS than that of deficient brush border cell enzymes. When you are actively involved in the elimination diet process, you have to be preoccupied with questioning the specific foods that you contemplate eating. In addition, you have to remain aware of how you physically feel and be alert concerning the progression of improvement in your general physical state and well-being.

The reason I am spending so much time on this aspect of eliminating the causative food offenders is that this is the key to self-diagnosing your specific pancreatic or intestinal enzyme insufficiencies. The quandary of the IBS or EPIEI (Exocrine Pancreatic Intestinal Enzyme Insufficiency) condition is due to a few main factors. One fairly common issue is that people tend not to discuss their condition with others and even fail to tell their doctors unless speaking to a gastroenterologist. This can arise out of intimidation, embarrassment, and frustration. IBS patients often feel beaten down by their discouragement, often feeling disillusioned, and tend to give up by succumbing to acceptance. At the same time, physicians usually feel equal frustration owing to the lack of a viable solution or treatment for IBS.

There are other considerations you need to keep in mind. During my own experience in dealing with my IBS during these past fifteen years, I became very aware and attuned to my body. Looking back on my condition, I noticed that my condition had gradually worsened over time. Unfortunately I cannot make a blanket statement by saying all patients will or do go through the same process. However, in view of my theory that IBS is an autoimmune response disease, a gradual deterioration and progressive demise of the brush border cells is quite plausible. When I first exhibited my symptoms, they were not as pronounced, and my ability to tolerate varied foods was not as compromised as it was a decade later. As my symptoms became more pronounced and my episodic tendencies increased, my diet became more restrictive. Ten years ago, I did not have a lactose intolerance issue. At the time, I consumed a lot of dairy. I loved cheeses of all varieties and yogurt, consumed butter, and enjoyed French cuisine.

If you take a step back and just think about this development, it will be easy to understand how my theory concerning EPIEI evolved. An interesting situation had arisen for me concerning a severe vitamin D and B deficiency. Eight years ago, I experienced lethargy and always felt tired. My lab work revealed that I had a severe vitamin D deficiency. My endocrinologist told me that he saw that a lot in diabetics, and I asked why this happened to me. He did not know the answer. I found out that there is a correlation between vitamin D deficiency and EPEI. The reason is that vitamin D is a fat-soluble vitamin. If you lack the enzyme to break down fat (i.e., lipase) then your body can't metabolize or utilize the vitamin D in your diet. Please note that in the appendix of this book, I have furnished references of published medical papers that reported on the incidence of pancreatitis in type 1 and type 2 diabetics. The occurrences of pancreatitis and EPIEI are high and are much more common in diabetics then endocrinologists and gastroenterologists are aware of. A medical paper published in

September 2014 discusses this in great detail. This condition has now been classified as type 3c diabetes.

Before leaving the discussion of Step I and the logging of your food intake along with bathroom progress, I should review the FODMAP diet. This will enable you to avoid offending foods in order to institute the intestinal lining healing process in preparation for ascertaining which enzymes are deficient via reintroduction of the offending foods one at a time.

List of High-FODMAP Foods That Must Be Avoided

Wheat-Based Foods

bread
cakes
pastries
biscuits
flour
batter
breadcrumbs / bread coatings
pasta
noodles
wheat- or bran-based cereals
crackers
crispbreads

Please note that the above foods should be replaced by gluten-free products.

Fruits to Avoid
apple
apricot

cherry

lychee

mango

nectarine

peach

pear

plum

prune

starfruit

watermelon

juices, sweets, or foods containing apple or pear juice

Avoid Most Nuts

Vegetables to Avoid

artichoke

asparagus

avocado

beans and pulses (baked beans, broad beans, butter beans, chick
peas, kidney beans, lentils)

beetroot

broccoli

brussels sprouts

cabbage

cauliflower

chicory root

fennel

garlic (including soups and sauces with added garlic)

leek

mange tout

mushroom

onion (including soups and sauces with added onion)

peas
onions
sugar snap peas

Dairy-Based Foods

Avoid all dairy-based foods and replace them with lactose-free milk, cheeses, yogurt, sour cream, cream cheese, and other lactose-free products.

Artificial Sweeteners

Absolutely do not use any artificial sweeteners, including the following:

fructose
high-fructose corn syrup
Fruisana
honey
isomalt
maltitol
mannitol
molasses
sorbitol
xylitol

High-FODMAP Food List (Avoid These Foods)

Fruits	Vegetables/Legumes	Nuts	Dairy	Sweeteners
apple	artichoke	almonds	*	**
apricot	asparagus	cashews		
blackberries	baked beans	pistachios		
boysenberries	broccoli			
cherries	brussels sprouts			
dates	cabbage			
figs	cauliflower			
mango	celery			
nectarine	fennel			
peaches	garlic			
pears	kidney beans			
persimmon	leeks			
plums	mushrooms			
prunes	onions			
watermelon	peas			
	pumpkin			
	soy beans			
dried fruits	snow peas			
fruit juices	sugar snap peas			

*　It is advisable to avoid all dairy until you are sure that you are not lactose intolerant.

**　Do not use any artificial sweeteners and limit plain sugar.

Additionally, do not consume foods containing inulin. Inulin is a polysaccharide and is found in onions, garlic, leeks and asparagus.

Low-FODMAP Food List (Acceptable Safe Foods)

Fruit	Vegetables	Dairy	Sweeteners
banana	alfalfa	*	**
blueberries	arugula		
cantaloupe	bamboo shoots		
clementine	bean sprouts		
cranberries	bell peppers		
grapes (limited)	bok choy		
grapefruit (limited)	butternut squash (limited)		
honeydew	carrots		
kiwi	chives		
lemon	corn (limited)		
lime	cucumber		
mandarin	endive		
orange	ginger		
passion fruit	green beans		
pineapple	kale		
raspberries	lettuce		
rhubarb	okra (limited)		
strawberries	olives		
tangelo	parsnip		
	potato		
	radish		
	red chili		
	silver beets		
	spinach		
	squash		
	sweet potato (limited)		
	tomato		
	turnip		
	water chestnuts		
	yams		
	zucchini		

*   Again, avoid dairy and use lactose-free products until you are sure that you are not lactose intolerant. After reassurance of being lactose free, still exercise limited consumption of dairy.

**   Please avoid all artificial sweeteners and fructose. Please limit your glucose intake.

*** Limit your nut consumption, and totally avoid nuts on the high-FODMAP list.

Additional, do not consume foods containing inulin. Inulin is a polysaccharide and is often extracted from chicory and is used as a food additive.

I am sure you are looking for time frames and guidelines regarding how long you have to conduct this elimination diet. The answer purely depends upon your physical condition and how much damage your mucosa or intestinal lining sustained from the repeated food insults. I will say it is purely guess work and depends upon how long you have been going through the damage/repair cycle. Past history has shown that the human body's ability to recover from an insult or damage does not always yield full recovery and that the length of time for recovery can take progressively longer after each incident.

Now that you understand the importance of keeping an accurate and detailed log of all of the foods you consume and your bathroom activities, you will observe patterns and the progression of the healing and repair of your intestinal lining. Please understand that every patient is different, as different enzyme-producing cells may have been compromised in each patient. If you were deficient in lipase, then your exocrine pancreatic acinar cells may have been compromised. Lipase is also produced to a lesser degree in your mouth and stomach. If that was an issue for you, it would be easy to tell by judging and observing your stool. If your stool floats and you can visibly see bubbles and or fat globules on the surface, then it would be a fair assumption that you are deficient in lipase and therefore can't digest fat.

As you approach day ten of maintaining a diet devoid of those foods on the FODMAP list, you should certainly start to see an abatement of your symptoms and marked improvement in your physical state. You are the only one who can judge whether your body has returned to normal. Just bear in mind that every person is different and every person's sustained damage is not the same. I did previously state that for people diagnosed with celiac disease, it can take one year to repair the damage done to the mucosal lining after removal of gluten from the diet. Some celiac patients achieve only a 70 percent repair of their brush border after five years of being gluten free. Honesty is an essential requirement to ensure that you do not cheat and short circuit this diagnostic procedure. Assuming that you have returned to normal, you can move to Step II.

Step II

Now that you are pain free and are no longer experiencing cramping, gas, bloating, or loose stools, you are ready to use those foods on the FODMAP avoidance list to see if they will elicit a distasteful response that produces gas, bloating, soreness, pain, or burning. On the other hand, if you now feel better and want to avoid returning to the pain, discomfort, and suffering, then you really do not have to perform the reintroduction of these foods, because you now know the answer and understand what really causes your IBS.

You have the option to remain on this draconian restrictive diet or you can live on a modified diet along with treatment that can offer a fair degree of relief and homeostasis. I might sound nebulous, and you might feel that I am not offering you a clear and concise resolution. The key here is the degree to which you are deficient in exocrine pancreatic enzymes or intestinal enzymes. Remember that some people can eat one or two slices of pizza but can't eat ice cream. Why? They are still producing some lactase to digest the milk sugar but not enough for a heavy load of lactose, such as that found in ice cream. The same scenario goes for the other enzymes that break down those sugars in the foods on the FODMAP diet that are to be avoided.

So is Step II reintroduction necessary? Not really if you are now able to understand how mildly or how severely your small intestine brush border cells have been compromised. This stage is trial and error.

When you start to reintroduce the foods on the avoid list, please do so in a slow and metered process. It is strongly suggested that you reintroduce only one forbidden food at a time, because otherwise you could overload your small intestines and cause a major breakdown of your mucosal lining. I can tell you from my own experience that if I sustain a minor insult from ingesting a small quantity of a forbidden fruit, I will recover in a day with minor discomfort. However, if I were to go to a Mexican restaurant and eat a large quantity of guacamole, it would take at least one week to ten days to effect a recovery. Remember: this is all about the haves and the have-nots. It is just dictated by the degree of damage to your brush border cells.

The next chapter will outline the treatment protocol. Before I discuss the method of treatment, I want to discuss three other conditions that might be connected to your EPIEI or IBS. I need to talk about lactose intolerance, SIBO, and gluten intolerance.

Lactose Intolerance

Lactose intolerance should now be easy for you to understand. We live in the United States, which makes us very fortunate, because we now have a full complement of lactose-free products for lactose-intolerant people. Contrary to what some medical theologians postulate—that lactose intolerance occurs because as adults we no longer need milk for our sustenance (in other words, because we no longer need mother's milk after we are weaned from our mothers)—the etiology of lactose intolerance falls under the umbrella of EPIEI (Exocrine Pancreatic Intestinal Enzyme Insufficiency). Remember that African Americans and Asian groups have a disproportionate amount of lactose-intolerant people. In all likelihood Ground zero for lactose intolerance is the ilium—the last part of your small intestine. This region has the highest population of brush border cells devoted to the production of lactase—the enzyme that breaks down the milk sugar molecule lactose. A very interesting consideration is that there is a large population of lactobacillus bacteria that reside in the ilium. The likelihood of a pathogen attacking the brush border cells responsible for lactase production is quite real. We can't discount an autoimmune predisposition either. Research needs to be commenced in this area. Just ask yourself how many people you know who have expressed feelings of discomfort after eating a rich meal containing cream sauces, desserts containing ice cream and whipped cream, or other dairy-laden rich foods. Those comments are often verbalized in passing without much thought or discussion. The person might exhibit a queasy, uncomfortable feeling that subsides without leaving much residual discomfort. Yet some exhibit full-blown symptoms of sharp pain, gas, bloating, and cramping. By now you know why these symptoms appear.

If you observe other cultures—such as the French, for example—view their culinary habits and lifestyles. Their daily lives consists of a steady diet of cheeses of every variety, cream sauces, butter and more butter, along with desserts laden with every dairy derivative. There goes the theory that the ability to produce lactase is a vestigial human function for lactose metabolism. One saving grace we have is the availability of over-the-counter lactase enzyme-replacement tablets, such as Lactaid, which can be purchased in retail grocery and drug stores. The ease of consuming one or more tablets with your first bite of lactose-containing foods can, in fact, prevent the usual discomfort one feels from lactose intolerance. Dosage is purely up to the patient. The lactose load is what dictates dosage. Please note that you cannot overdose on lactase. Any excess lactase is harmless and is metabolized by your body. Lactase is an enzyme, which is a protein that is normally produced by your body. Remember that an enzyme is just a catalyst that helps bring about or start a reaction (e.g., the breakdown of lactose [milk sugar]).

This means that dispensing is up to you. My advice is to be generous with dispensing of the Lactaid tablets. The larger the dairy or lactose content of the meal, the more tablets you should ingest. If it's a lot of cheese pizza, then take a tablet at the first bite and another with each successive piece. This all is predicated upon the severity of your lactose intolerance or enzyme deficiency. An example is that I am on the high end of being lactose intolerant, so when I eat just two ounces of aged cheddar cheese, I need a minimum of four Lactaid tablets to avoid symptoms and discomfort. Each person is different and must judge their situation accordingly.

It is important to note that medicine is aware of temporary situations of lactose intolerance. This condition is not entirely uncommon for a patient who presents with a severe viral or bacterial intestinal infection, such as what is commonly called a stomach flu. Naturally, the reason for this outcome is due to the destruction of the brush border cells within the small intestine that produce lactase. Without the lactase enzyme present after infection, the patient cannot digest dairy products. In most instances, the brush border does repair itself and regenerate the cells necessary to produce lactase enzyme again after the recovery from the sustained infection. It can take a few months for repair and restoration. This is termed PILI (Post infectious lactose intolerance).

Of course those patients that sustain permanent damage will remain lactose intolerant for the rest of their lives if their enzyme-producing brush border cells cannot regenerate. This simple fact is support for my theory on the cause of IBS. The theory that I have stated is much more complex and has a varied basis for the development of IBS. The essence here is that selective destruction of specific enzyme-producing brush border cells can contribute to the etiology of IBS. Again, the degree of an individual's IBS is related to the degree of damage of his or her enzyme-producing brush border cells. This also encompasses exocrine pancreatic digestive enzymes.

SIBO (Small Intestinal Bacterial Overgrowth)

If you ever have been diagnosed with SIBO, then you understand the symptoms. Are they in fact the same as those present in EPIEI or IBS? Of course it is a sad truth that the attending physician cannot offer you the etiology. The form of treatment offered is a round of antibiotics, namely Xifaxan, which is prescribed as the solution. When a patient asks what the cause is, the physician will respond, "Well, we don't know, but this antibiotic controls the infection." Is that really the answer? Of course not. The age-old story of physicians treating the symptoms and not the cause comes into play here.

In earlier sections of this book, I discussed this in detail. I also paraphrased studies done on type 1 and type 2 diabetics, and I even reported on a new classification of diabetes—type 3c diabetes. A type 3c diabetic exhibits EPIEI. Oh, how interesting! I also discussed the high incidence of SIBO in both type 1 and type 2 diabetics. Gee, do you think autoimmune response disease comes into play here? Maybe just like diabetes? Of course you now realize why. My theory is based on the fact that the explosive bacterial overgrowth is due to a patient's IEI (Intestinal Enzyme Insufficiency) and a minor degree of PEI (Pancreatic Enzyme Insufficiency). Without the presence of the enzymes to break down those large complex sugars, you provide an excessive amount of an unnatural food supply for the residential bacteria.

Bear in mind that SIBO is not only relegated to diabetics, and it would be safe to assume that patients who suffer from EPIEI can easily develop SIBO. Since I am not a physician, I cannot state that SIBO should not be treated with antibiotics. In view of the suggested policies on the usage of antibiotics in the United States, the policies of the Centers for Disease Control (CDC) and the National Institutes of Health (NIH) advise restraint in overprescribing antibiotics. Overprescription and overuse of antibiotics helps create bacteria resistant to antibiotics, thereby reducing the effectiveness of our current antibiotics. It is much more prudent to reduce the food source of the residential bacteria in the intestines by preventing the presence of the overabundance of large, complex undigested sugars due to EPIEI. An interesting note is that I have not had a reoccurrence of SIBO since starting my treatment protocol for my EPIEI, and I no longer exhibit those past symptoms. Therefore, it is safe to say that I no longer have SIBO. The obvious reason is that, being on my treatment protocol, I no longer have undigested large complex sugar molecules in my duodenum, jejunum, or ilium that would facilitate an explosive overgrowth of bacteria. When considering the variation among the resident intestinal bacteria, one can assume that homeostasis is normally maintained between the varied bacterial species. It is when a specific species, such as a lactobacillus pathogen, gains advantage via the overabundance of excess sugars that SIBO results. This is not a proven fact, but it is quite plausible.

Gluten Intolerance

This subject is, without doubt, a hot potato, and you will enjoy becoming enlightened. I published an article on gluten and type 2 diabetes. This can provide good insight into the quandary of the current gluten argument.

Commentary: November 13, 2013

By: Lawrence Bodner

Why are we experiencing a type 2 diabetes epidemic today, and what is the gluten connection? The answer is simple and obvious. If we look at societal and cultural changes that occurred during the last forty years in the United States, we can easily comprehend how this epidemic materialized. A *New York Times* article by Sendhil Mullainthan from November 10, 2013, titled "The Co-Villains Behind Obesity's Rise" provides scientific explanation and theory.

In plain and simple language, we are eating ourselves to death, exporting our societal cultural shift in dietary habits, and causing major self-directed epidemics of disease. Unfortunately there is not one simple causative agent but rather many factors that encompass lifestyle and the quantity and ingredients of modern-day twenty-first-century American food.

Let us take a brief tour over the last hundred years of American cultural and societal changes. As a nation, we went from an agrarian society where a major segment of our population farmed, the rest of the population worked physically in factories, and women worked physically in the home, performing household chores without modern-day conveniences. One hundred years ago, we consumed calories that were metabolized (burned up) by hard physical labor.

In addition, the American food industry was in its infancy, and a majority of Americans consumed their meals at home. The home-cooked meals were wholesome and were made from unprocessed natural ingredients.

Just take breads for example. Toward the end of the nineteenth century, breads were baked at home along with other baked goods. There were bakeries, but those few bakeries baked in the same fashion as that of the homemaker. In the middle to late 1800s, white bleached flower came on the scene. This was the initial blow to good health. Bleached flour removed the germ (the outer layer of the wheat grain), all of the gluten, vitamins, and nutrients. This process was created because the whole grains spoiled and rotted quickly after milling, and when the railroad came on the scene, the grains were valueless and had no nutritional value by the time they reached their destination. This new flour required the reintroduction of gluten to give the flour back its elastic consistency, as well as the reintroduction of vitamins and minerals. This process in turn resulted in excessive gluten in the flour. This is a likely cause of modern-day gluten intolerance. Bear in mind that this change occurred very slowly and the American culinary culture still adhered to the same habits in most cities. This was a very gradual shift.

Why is this factor so important? This was the first retreat from natural, wholesome, and healthy foods. Please don't think this change occurred overnight. Most bakers and homemakers still baked breads in the old-fashioned tradition by using natural grains and letting the dough slowly rise and cure. This also metabolized the gluten.

Now we will fast forward to 2010. Americans no longer eat whole grains, unprocessed foods, or foods without additives and chemicals. One hundred years ago, only small corner grocers existed alongside neighboring butcher shops, fruit and produce shops, and bakeries all selling fresh, unprocessed foods. At that time, fast food did not exist; neither did the processed snack foods that take up multiple aisles in our supermarkets today. Do you comprehend what occurred? On a metabolic level, our societal and cultural changes influenced the way we metabolize the new food style. Unfortunately, this whole obesity, diabesity, and type 2 diabetes epidemic is complex, making it difficult to understand. Medical professionals, researchers, and lay people can be quick to accuse and surmise that genetics is the root cause.

I beg to differ. Just study societal and cultural changes that have occurred worldwide in the last two decades. Look at emerging third-world countries, such as Vietnam. As the United States became aggressive in the export of her culture and fast food retail chains, type 2 diabetes exploded in Europe, Asia, and South America. So why did this occur in the last fifty years? Although white flour existed for a long time, fast food; huge varieties of snack foods laden with sugar, fat, and added gluten; and supersized portions pushed our bodies over the line into compromised health.

Here is the easy overview explanation. One hundred years ago, our foods had a complex composition that required a slow metabolic process to break down the food. Now the food is preprocessed, using white bleached flour with numerous additives including, but not limited to, sugar, high fructose corn sweetener, and added gluten. This in turn also helped produce a new health crisis called metabolic syndrome. Metabolic syndrome is the presence of central obesity, hyperglycemia, hypertension, and hyperlipidemia (high blood sugar, high blood pressure, and elevated blood fats), which all present at the same time in the patient.

The search for the cause of gluten intolerance is still in the investigative stage at the time of this publication. The important thing is to understand why there has been an increase in the amount of Americans that complain of or exhibit symptoms of gluten intolerance. One word that certainly comes to mind is "excess." Half a century ago, excess gluten was not in our diets in the proportions it is today. The gluten molecule is a very large molecule and can present issues in your small intestine in terms of digestion and permeability across the intestinal wall. Without devoting an excessive amount of time, I will just mention one observation of my youth. When I was a preteen, our new grocery store—not yet a supermarket—had just one or two types of bags of chips and pretzels, and a few varieties of cookies, crackers, and snacks. They contained simple, limited ingredients. Today when you read a food label, it is akin to reading a short novel. Also, the presence of obesity was essentially nonexistent in the 1950s. When I attended grade school, middle school, and high school, we rarely observed obesity and rarely had overweight schoolmates.

One interesting observation is that people who have removed gluten from their diet have noticed that their huger abated and they lost weight after becoming gluten free.

Why does excessive gluten cause excessive weight gain and type 2 diabetes? Complex foods are not normally metabolized in the mouth. Our food is just initially masticated and bathed in saliva, and it receives amylase in the mouth to prepare it for the stomach. Highly processed foods, such as white flour, are initially broken down into sugars when they enter the mouth. Your saliva begins to break down the white flour, and the sugars get dumped directly into your bloodstream, circumventing the stomach and regular metabolism. Excessive consumption causes a spike in your blood sugar. In addition, if your body does not need the calories, then your liver converts the glucose to glycogen and your body stores it as fat. Hence, we become fat if our bodies do not burn the newly stored fat deposits.

This brings me to lifestyle. We no long perform physical labor, and our children no longer engage in physical play outside. We replaced those activities with office work, computer usage, digital games, PDAs, television, and a generally sedentary lifestyle. That was the setup for type 2 diabetes. Chances are that a small segment of the population had a propensity toward type 2 diabetes but it did not manifest itself because we did not exceed optimal weight and our pancreases produced enough insulin. By the way, type 2 diabetes can also be caused by insulin resistance. Exercise does aid in getting the insulin molecules produced in the pancreas through the bloodstream and into the individual cells. You need insulin to get the glucose into each cell for cell metabolism. Glucose is the fuel for our cells.

If you doubt any of this, then look at countries that are growing and transforming from third-world to second- and first-world countries. Vietnam, China, India, Japan, Korea, and many other countries are experiencing diabetes epidemics as their countries see major migrations of large segments of their populations from the farms and rice paddies to the cities, which now have McDonalds, Burger King, Dunkin' Doughnuts, Kentucky Fried Chicken, and more. Their diets went from rice and fish to fried and fast foods, sugar, gluten, high-fructose corn syrup, and fat-laden foods. A sad result of this is that Vietnam now has the highest rate of amputations in the world, which is purely due to their type 2 diabetes epidemic.

If one does not grasp all of the above, just remember four words: content, quantity, frequency, and exercise. This will be your key to controlling weight gain, obesity, type 2 diabetes, and metabolic syndrome.

The above commentary is a broad overview of a cataclysmic shift that is occurring throughout the world today. This crisis and the result of it are usually explained as having a medical origin or predisposition. If that were, in fact, the case, then why did prediabetes and type 2 diabetes not present in pediatrics before 1992? I can almost assign the label "a disease of choice" to type 2 diabetes.

One other topic to discuss in relation to gluten intolerance is gluten sensitivity. Recent studies have correlated gluten sensitivity to the condition called leaky gut syndrome. Remember that your intestinal lining is composed of a single layer of enterocyte cells that normally form a tight barrier for your intestines. When we discuss gluten, we must look at gliadin, zonulin, and lectin. There is no question that gluten sensitivity can play a role in IBS. Gliadin is a protein that gives wheat its doughy consistency, and when consumed in excess it can stimulate your brush border cells to produce zonulin. This intestinal protein can stimulate your body to open the spaces between the enterocyte cells that form the single-layer lining of your intestine (gut). Hence, we develop leaky gut syndrome. Stimulating open gaps between the enterocyte cells allows permeability and permits nutrients, toxins, and wastes to easily flow from your intestines into your bloodstream and surrounding tissues. This in turn causes an immune response that results in inflammation.

Lectin is a naturally occurring protein in grain seeds that protects the seeds against predator insects and other opportunists seeking food. This is present in wheat germ, and our diets have been expanding our usage of wheat germ. Remember the word "excess," because humans love to do everything in excess! Over the last century, and particularly within the last forty years, we have supersized our appetites, diets, and bodies. In turn, we have been consuming excess amounts of gluten, sugars, and processed foods, which have all created modern-day medical problems and issues of gluten intolerance, gluten sensitivity, IBS, type 2 diabetes, leaky gut syndrome, and inflammatory bowel disease.

The age-old question is "Are we to blame for this crisis? The answer is "Only partially." I say that because adults and children alike have fallen victim to secrets held by food manufacturers. I have discussed how our society metamorphosed from an agrarian society to an industrialized society to a modern-day digitized society. Our food preparation and eating habits changed too. We went from home cooking utilizing slow natural cooking processes to commercialized and industrialized processed foods. Over these last three decades, consumers have experienced the introduction of trans fats (which has now been removed from foods), adulterated gluten added to most food products, high-fructose corn syrup, cane juice, sucrose, and numerous other additives that have taxed our bodies. Many of these additives play havoc on children and adults alike. The incredible amounts of sugars we consume daily has exerted a tremendous toll on our society, fostering markedly increased obesity. The amounts of sugar, high-fructose corn syrup, and sucrose in sodas that children drink daily add to increased obesity, type 2 diabetes, and hyperactivity. The added gluten in snacks, cookies, breads, waffles, pretzels, and numerous other foods induces us to want more and eat more. Excess gluten increases appetite. Although the food industry has a right to produce and market their products, our society has the obligation to ensure the safety and well-being of its citizens. Labeling containing explanations and risks should be required.

In conclusion, when we address a complex problem, such as the metabolic crisis that I have been discussing, we are always looking for a short and concise answer. One phrase comes to my mind, and that is "Supersize it." That phrase says it all. The real question is, did the public demand it, or did the food industry create the demand by increasing the sizes, portions, and contents of the food products they market, create, and sell? Science and medicine function on empirical research, studies, and supportive factual documentation. Yet if we look at this worldwide crisis through the eyes of a sociologist, a historian, and a behavioral psychologist, it is not too hard to see how this metabolic epidemic metamorphosed into a medical crisis.

When we study medicine, we realize that the human body is forgiving—but only to a certain point. If a body exhibits blood markers that are temporarily out of range and return to normal, then the body can possibly avoid permanent damage or change from the short duration of an abnormal situation. It is when we push our bodies to the limit by inflicting radical change, such as morbid obesity for a sustained period of time, that we invite multiple morbidity (many medical conditions). We must be honest and clear here in order to see the etiologies and reasons for these modern-day medical conditions.

I have stated throughout this book that I believe in a genetic predisposition for EPIEI (Exocrine Pancreatic Intestinal Enzyme Insufficiency). However, regarding gluten intolerance and other digestive diseases, lifestyle changes and abusive excesses in diet can exert outside influences. This concept is considered in understanding cancer. Basically what I am discussing is the relationship of external influences and insults, which can be labeled as "acquired" as opposed to "inherited." Does this mean that if a person has a genetic or inherited predisposition for cancer, an acquired situation—such as a toxic stressor like an environmental carcinogen—can play a role in developing a cancer? It most assuredly does. And a significant portion of the development of type 2 diabetes and a degree of gluten intolerance can follow in the same fashion. The word is "excess." A poison or toxin will not kill you in minute or trace amounts, but a large quantity will. The same goes for excessive eating of carbohydrates, sugar, fructose, gluten, etc.

When you try to understand what happened in the last half century and you see the radical cataclysmic shift that occurred in our diets and our increases in weight and girth, you must ask why this happened.

The answer is the food industry, but I will not place all of the blame on the food manufacturers. The public at large makes the choice to buy their products. The unfortunate byproduct of the industry's radical change in food composition was increased desire for the newly produced highly processed foods. Another issue is the gluten. If you read labels on products today, you will find that gluten is added to a majority of food products. This overload of gluten increases appetite and desire for more. Now you know why we are rapidly becoming an obese society and why we experience such an increase of IBS, leaky gut syndrome, and gluten intolerance and sensitivity, along with the explosive growth of type 2 diabetes.

If we fail to address this crisis, it could, in fact, bankrupt our country with its undue burden on our health care system. Without doing historical research, I would assume that in all probability IBS and gluten intolerance was not as pronounced in the general population one hundred years ago as it is today. In closing, I hope you have attained a broad knowledge of digestion. This will clearly aid you in understanding how to treat your EPIEI.

CHAPTER 9

How to Use the Treatment Protocol for EPIEI (Exocrine Pancreatic Intestinal Enzyme Insufficiency)

In starting to discuss my treatment protocol for EPIEI, I can frankly say that my condition has improved by almost 95 percent. That means that I very rarely experience any symptoms. The most important consideration that you must understand is that each patient who presents with EPIEI is not the same. There are two considerations that must be addressed. Clearly understand that out of the digestive enzymes that we discussed, not all are deficient in a patient. Furthermore, each patient can vary as to whether he or she is deficient in one or more pancreatic enzymes, in intestinal (brush border) enzymes, or a combination thereof. On top of this complexity, every patient can vary in his or her degree of being compromised or deficient. So how do we know which enzyme-replacement therapy should be prescribed and how much should be dosed? Let me talk about that.

First of all, I must be clear here. I am not a physician, and I am not prescribing a pharmaceutical. The enzyme-replacement therapy is not an FDA-controlled medication and is considered a supplement. I want you to understand this explanation in order to alleviate any fears that you might have about taking enzyme-replacement therapy. Remember that an enzyme is a catalyst and is protein based. Therefore, it does not become part of the reaction of the chemical process of breaking down a food component such as a complex sugar; rather, it starts the reaction. The second consideration is that since it is a protein and not a drug or unnatural substance, you cannot overdose on enzyme-replacement therapy. Any excess that is not needed after ingestion will be processed like any other protein-based food without harm.

There are a few reasons that an effective treatment protocol for enzyme-replacement therapy for EPIEI has not been formulated, established, and developed to date. The failure of diagnosis of the condition and understanding of its etiology compromised the ability of the practitioner to treat the disease. That is why labels such as "IBS" and "malabsorption" were used.

It is important to understand that when you cruise through the aisles of grocery stores, vitamin shops, health-food stores, and Internet websites for supplements, the greatest consideration you should give is to the units of each enzyme contained in each capsule. Cost is always the manufacturer's concern. Important enzymes are expensive and are added in trace amounts in an inexpensive product. Also important is the way the product is formulated. If the capsule is not coated with an enteric, then in all likelihood the enzymatic contents will be destroyed by stomach acid. As you read further, you will see that the ERT (Enzyme Replacement Therapy) mentioned here is coated with an enteric and contains the proper amount and concentration of the necessary ERT.

Please note that I am not criticizing physicians for their failure to understand the condition of EPIEI. I discovered the etiology of EPIEI through an unanticipated accidental reaction to chemotherapy. I was fortunate that I was able to carefully study and analyze my own condition and through extensive research by reading available published medical papers, reading presentations at international gastroenterology medical conventions, reading published veterinary medicine papers on pancreatitis, and reading research on disease causing damage to the brush borders of rabbits and rats that clearly displayed resultant intestinal enzyme insufficiencies. This enabled me to formulate my theory. It is very fair to assume that if I were not on the GM-CSF for my melanoma, and if I did not have a predisposition for autoimmune disease as in my type 1 diabetes, I would never have established the correlation between EPIEI and predisposed autoimmune disease.

How Do I Start My Enzyme-Replacement Therapy?

Straight-out, I will tell you that we must commence with a shotgun approach. Now that you understand the mechanics, chemistry, and actions of digestion, you can understand why I chose this approach. Two considerations come into play here. The first consideration is that we are dealing with the feasibility of being deficient in one or more of the digestive enzymes. The second consideration is that current medicine has not devised effective and minimally invasive diagnostic testing to detect your specific enzyme insufficiency other than in the case of the aftermath of pancreatitis. Therefore, the responsibility rests in your lap. Through the elimination diet, you have hopefully narrowed down the offending food or food groups that are the causative agents. Through this process you will then able to figure out which EPIEs you are deficient in. You, the patient, are the only one who can detect the degree and severity of a reaction to an offending food. Your effective treatment protocol depends on the length of time that you have had EPIEI and your ability to observe.

Let's start now.

There are four steps to this treatment.

1. Determine whether or not you either have hyperacidity or
    suffer from acid reflux. If either condition applies to you, then
    you must take an antacid before you take your ERT to avoid
    destruction of the ERT in excessive stomach acid.
2. Think about what food or meal you are about to eat.
    a) Mexican food: beans, avocado, onions, sour cream,
        cheese
    c) French food: cheese, butter, dairy, onions, shallots, cream
    d) A buffet: watermelon, peaches, apples, cherries,
        blackberries, mangoes, pears, plums
    b) Grilled marbled steak smothered in onions, garlic powder,
        garlic cloves, salad (red onions, tomatoes, artichoke,
        garlic olive oil dressing), a side of fettuccine with cream
        and butter sauce, zucchini
    e) lamb chops, onions, garlic, buttered potatoes, creamed
        spinach
    f) When you look at the above list, what stands out to
        you? If you are lactose intolerant then it was a flashing
        red light to you when you read a, b, d, and e. Therefore,
        whether eating at home or out, you must be armed with
        Lactaid brand lactase tablets. Treatment before meals
        containing dairy (ingesting Lactaid tablets before your
        first bite of dairy-containing foods) will prevent lactose
        intolerance symptoms from developing. Each dose is
        temporary and is only for the current meal that you
        eat. You cannot overdose on Lactase enzyme! Therefore,
        taking large doses rather than underdosing is strongly
        advisable until you develop an understanding of your
        specific degree of lactose intolerance (lactase production

deficiency in your intestinal brush border cells). Please note that Lactaid brand lactase tablets are individually foil wrapped and conveniently sold over the counter in supermarkets and drugstores. They are usually available in the vitamin and supplement aisle. Make sure you always have an ample supply in a purse or pocket. My advice is that if you are severely lactose intolerant, you should take the tablet before the first bite, several during the meal, and one after the last bite.

If you are not sure if you are lactose intolerant, then just review the symptoms. Think about whether you develop sharp pain or a funny feeling of discomfort in your abdomen about twenty minutes after eating cheese, ice cream, butter, cheese pizza, pasta with cheese filling, etc. Do you develop gas, bloating, cramping, pain, and subsequent lose stools later? If you answer yes, then you are more than likely lactose intolerant. If you are currently feeling normal and symptom free now, consider taking Lactaid tablets before your next meal of a dairy-based food in order to see if it works for you. Depending upon your degree of symptoms, supplement accordingly. This means that if you suffer minor discomfort, then you can supplement sparingly. If you suffer severe symptoms, then supplement liberally. This means you can take as much Lactaid as is needed to accommodate the amount of cheese or other dairy you consume. You cannot overdose with lactase. Just remember that there is a full range of lactose-free dairy products available today, and so this treatment might just be relegated to occasional meals at home for which a lactose-free ingredient is not available. Otherwise it will be useful for eating out in restaurants and at other people's homes. When in doubt, use Lactaid if you suspect, but are not sure, that a restaurant meal contains ingredients such as butter, cheese, or cream.

We now must consider list items c, d, and e. Here we are going to address the complex sugars in fruits, onions, garlic, and artichoke, and then we will also address the fat from the steak and lamb chops.

The term IBS is so broad and undefined because the symptoms, degree of severity, and its inconsistency are so expansive that medicine never developed a clear diagnosis, etiology, or form of treatment for the disease. I am without doubt an extreme example of a patient with a broad range of EPIEIs. I can clearly tell you that I am not deficient in lipase, the enzyme that initiates fat metabolism, but I do probably underproduce lipase, because I present with a vitamin D deficiency. I do not present with symptoms of inability to metabolize fat, but in truth my diet has minor fat content, most of which is not derived from animal fat. After intensive study, observation, and trial and error, I was able to deduce what exocrine pancreatic intestinal enzymes I am deficient in. The reason I am discussing my case is to provide you with an understanding of how I treat my particular condition and why.

In 2014, I reached maximum frustration because I was approaching my fifteenth year of suffering with no relief other than the recovery periods between severe gastrointestinal distress. At the time, I did not realize that I was unconsciously effecting a healing process because I lacked a desire to eat the offending foods after each progressive episode. By temporarily eliminating the offenders, I allowed my mucosal intestinal lining to repair and heal. I can clearly tell you that each successive year, that task became more difficult and took longer. I surmise that my autoimmune response action to pathogenic bacteria caused my brush border glandular enzyme-producing cells in my small intestine's villi to become gradually compromised. This is an important logical theory.

Let me take a moment to discuss this. When I say "compromised," I am referring to a reduction in the presence of existing brush border enzyme-producing cells. You might not realize it, but this does occur in other areas of human anatomy. You might be more familiar with the human aging process. Have you ever asked yourself why older women often overuse perfume to the extent of almost taking a bath in the fragrance? How about people who have lost their sense of taste or sense of smell? I could go into hearing loss, but the loss of hearing is more involved and can have neurological causes, anatomical causes, and other complexities. Nonetheless, such desensitization can be caused by the loss of sensory cells, such as taste buds on the tongue or olfactory sensory cells in the nose. Also, it is important to understand that the senses of smell and taste are interconnected.

As you can see, the loss of active sensory cells or exocrine pancreatic and intestinal enzyme-producing cells can have a devastating effect on the health and well-being of an individual in each given situation. Think about the loss in numbers. By that I mean that the degree of loss of sense of taste, loss of sense of smell, and loss of exocrine and intestinal enzyme production all dictate the degree of severity, intensity, and loss of effectiveness.

At this point you might say, "Enough already! Let's get on with it! How do I treat myself?" I'm not trying to drag this out. My purpose is to set you up to understand how to treat yourself, how to derive the right dosage, and how to figure out which enzymes you are deficient in.

You will be treating your condition with two different ERTs. One will be exocrine pancreatic enzymes, and the other will be intestinal enzymes—mainly alpha-galactosidase. After months of trial and error, I figured out the dosage required for each meal, which enzyme replacement to take for the specific meal, and how to take it. Remember that Lactaid is lactase, which is also an ERT.

As you go through the titration stage—that is, the stage of figuring out the dosages you specifically require based on your particular deficiencies and based on the degree of severity of your lack of enzyme production—you will attain a proper treatment protocol. I can honestly say with absolute pleasure that I no longer exhibit frequent bowel movements, gas, bloating, pain, intestinal lining soreness, soft stools, urgency, or any other symptom.

On the next three pages, I have listed the enzyme-replacement products that I recommend. You will be using either Digest Gold or Xymogen's XymoZyme for broad-spectrum enzyme-replacement therapy, and you will be using Bean-zyme for additional coverage with alpha-galactosidase for the process of breaking down complex sugars. These three products are available on website portals, and I have provided the URL Internet addresses for you to purchase them on the Internet on the following three pages.

Digest Gold™ +PROBIOTICS

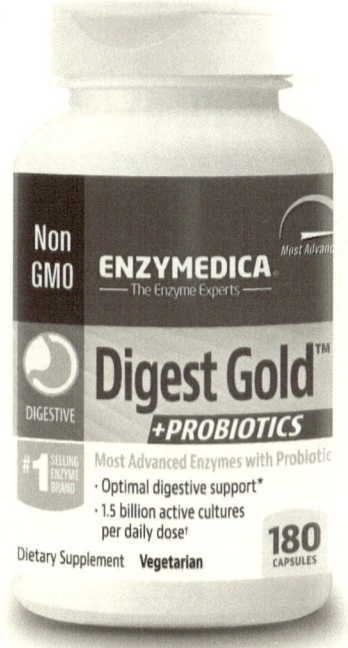

Supplement Facts		
Serving Size 1 Capsule		
Servings Per Container: 180		
Amount Per Serving		%DV
Amylase *Thera-blend*™	23,000 DU	**
Protease *Thera-blend*™	80,000 HUT	**
Glucoamylase	50 AGU	**
Alpha Galactosidase	450 GalU	**
Cellulase *Thera-blend*™	3,000 CU	**
Lipase *Thera-blend*™	4,000 FCCFIP	**
Lactase	900 ALU	**
Beta Glucanase	25 BGU	**
Maltase	200 DP°	**
Xylanase	550 XU	**
Pectinase (w/ Phytase)	45 Endo-PGU	**
Invertase	240 SU	**
Hemicellulase	30 HCU	**
Probiotic Blend:	500 million CFU	
L. acidophilus DDS-1, L. rhamnosus, L. casei, L. gasseri, L. plantarum, L. bulgaricus, L. salivarius, L. paracasei		

**Daily Value not established

OTHER INGREDIENTS: 100% Vegetarian Capsule (cellulose, water).
CONTAINS NO egg, dairy, preservatives, salt, sucrose, soy, wheat, yeast, nuts, corn, gluten, casein, potato, rice, artificial colors or flavors. **Keep closed in dry place; avoid excessive heat.**

Do not use if safety seal is broken or missing.
Enzymedica does not use ingredients produced using biotechnology.

This product is extensively available on many websites. Amazon.com offers many choices of vendors that carry this product.

Company website: www.enzymedica.com
Phone: 888-918-1118

XymoZyme

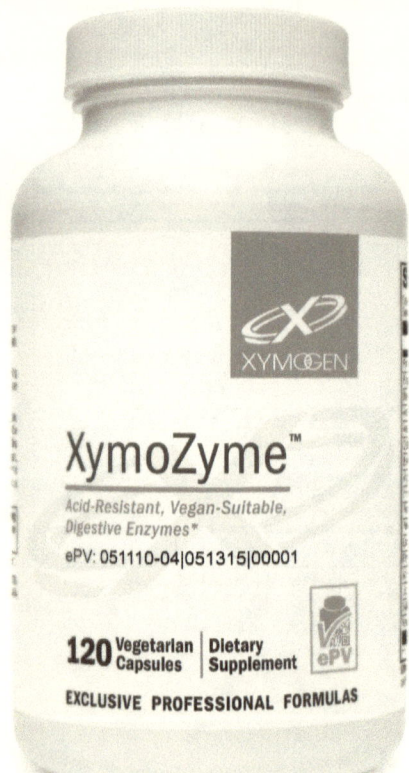

Supplement Facts

Serving Size: 2 Capsules
Servings Per Container: 60

	Amount Per Serving	%DV
Protease (pH 3.0-9.0)	120,000 HUT	**
Papain (from papaya)	50,000 TU	**
Bromelain (from pineapple)	120 GDU	**
Amylase	4,000 SKB	**
Amyloglucosidase (glucoamylase)	30 AG	**
Cellulase	4,000 CU	**
Beta-Glucanase	50 BGU	**
Alpha-Galactosidase	400 GAL	**
Invertase	2,000 Sumner	**
Peptidase (29 DPPIV)	2,400 HUT	**
Pectinase	70 Endo PG	**
Lactase	700 ALU	**
Phytase	20 U	**
Acid Stable Protease (pH 2.0-3.5)	400 HUT	**
Lipase	1,200 FIP	**
Xylanase	300 XU	**
Hemicellulase	200 HCU	**

**Daily Value (DV) not established.

Other Ingredients: HPMC (capsule), microcrystalline cellulose, stearic acid, magnesium stearate, and silica.

Company website: www.xymogen.com
Phone: 800-647-6100

Bean-zyme

Contents: alpha-galactosidase enzyme 300 GALU per dose (two capsules)

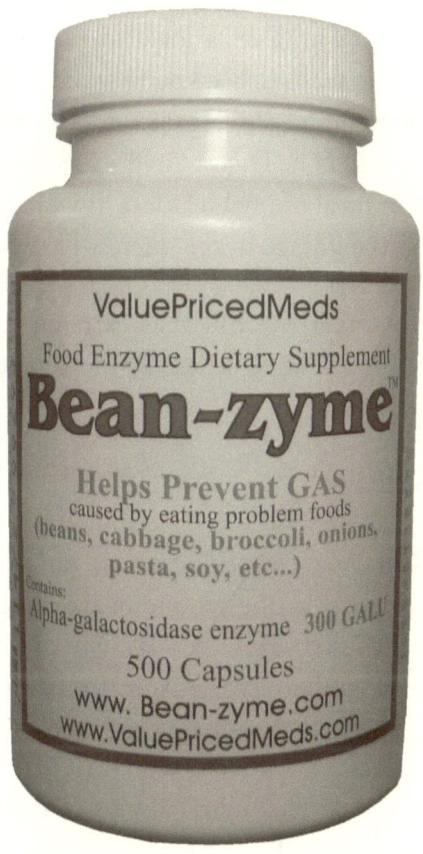

Company website: www.valuepricedmeds.com
Phone: 805-560-8369

Before you begin treatment, I assume that if you are lactose intolerant, you adjusted your dairy intake by replacing all dairy components of your diet with lactose-free dairy products.

Breakfast

In my particular situation, I eat a lot of fruit. Some of the fruit is on the offending list, such as blackberries and fruit preserves, so I take four Bean-zyme brand alpha-galactosidase capsules at the first ingestion of the fruit and one Digest Gold + Probiotics brand capsules when I eat the main meal of my breakfast. It works so well that I am fearful of reducing the dosage in the interest of cost savings.

Please bear in mind that my EPIEI is extreme, and therefore my treatment protocol might be significantly more aggressive than what you might require.

Midmorning Snacks

I am an insulin-dependent type 1 diabetic on an insulin infusion pump, and therefore my eating requirements consist of three main meals and three scheduled snacks per day. My snacks usually consist of lactose-free cheese and a piece of fruit. I take two Digest Gold + Probiotics brand capsules before eating the snack.

No matter where I am or what I do, I always carry four Tums tablets, at least six Digest Gold + Probiotics brand capsules, and a dozen Bran-zyme brand alpha-galactosidase capsules in a small tube. With this habit, I am always prepared no matter where I am. In addition, I keep Lactaid tablets in the car for the eventuality that I might eat out in a restaurant and forget my Lactaid at home.

Lunch

My lunch usually consists of cottage cheese or lactose-free yogurt; fruit, including melon, bananas, and berries; and walnuts. At the start of the meal, I take two Digest Gold + Probiotics brand capsules.

Snack

My afternoon snack might be a homemade dessert that my wife made, which contains fruit with a cheese component and might also have margarine in the crust. The ingredients are lactose free and gluten free but nonetheless contain many sugars that might be on the avoidance list. I always take one Digest Gold + Probiotics brand capsule, and if there are offending complex sugars, I will also take one or two Bean-zyme brand alpha-galactosidase capsules, even though Digest Gold contains alpha-galactosidase, for added protection.

Dinner

Before my first bite of salad, I start with the ingestion of four Bean-zyme brand alpha-galactosidase capsules. My dinner usually starts with a salad that often has avocado slices, sometimes strawberries, dried cranberries, walnuts, and standard greens. I rarely eat tomatoes and never eat onions or garlic even if I can correct with Bean-zyme brand alpha-galactosidase. For me it is just not worth the risk of an insult to my mucosal intestinal lining.

When I start my main course or entrée I always take two Digest Gold + Probiotics brand capsules. If the meal is in a restaurant setting, such as an Indian restaurant, I will be generous and dispense Bean-zyme brand alpha-galactosidase throughout the meal to cover myself for possible onions, garlic, and other seasonings that might be troublesome.

Bedtime Snack

Being an insulin-dependent diabetic, I must eat a snack before bed
to prevent a low blood sugar during the night. I still always take one
Digest Gold + Probiotics brand capsule before eating the snack.

Finding Your Own Treatment Protocol

Now that you see how I dispense the ERT, I must bring to your
attention that my treatment protocol is not a standard for universal
treatment. The nature of IBS or EPIEI is inconsistent, the degree of
severity varies from patient to patient, the specific enzyme deficiencies
vary from patient to patient, and the etiology varies too. Nonetheless,
the end result is that an EPIEI patient needs a unique treatment
protocol that is tailored to the patient's deficiencies.

It is up to you, the patient to figure out the degree of the severity of EPIEI
that you present with and the amount and type of ERT you require.
This can be achieved only by your desire to alleviate your discomfort
and suffering through your vigilance to figure out which EPIEs you are
deficient in and to titrate your specific requirements for your need for ERT.

Please feel confident that you cannot overdose on the enzyme
replacements discussed here that are contained in Digest Gold,
Xymogen-Xymozyme, Bean-zyme, and Lactaid branded ERTs.

If your doctor is perchance knowledgeable regarding this theory and is
aware of this treatment protocol, then he or she might be of assistance
to you. I hope I was clear in explaining the treatment protocol. The
reason I stated that the choice of the ERT is a shotgun approach is that
I have included all possible enzymes that might prove to be deficient.
It is similar in fashion to an antibiotic that is considered to be a broad-
spectrum drug. That means that it can treat a full range of bacterial
pathogens from gram-positive to gram-negative bacteria. Since we do

not know which EPIE you might be deficient in, I chose to treat most deficiencies. The nature of food preparation is that there are always unsuspected ingredients in a prepared meal unless you yourself are the one preparing from raw, unprocessed ingredients.

The ERTs that are available to the general public are listed on the preceding pages. In terms of contents and concentrations, you can view the therapy treatments listed on the accompanying charts. The enzyme contents and the quantities of each enzyme are detailed on the preceding pages.

Please note that I strongly advocate that you discuss this approach with your physician and ensure that there is not another medical reason for your condition!

I additionally use Bean-zyme for complex sugars contained in fruits, vegetables, preserves, jams, juices, candies, and desserts that present major issues because I do not produce alpha-galactosidase. This therapy is useful for situations where the offending food is relegated to fruits, vegetables, desserts, juices, jams, and candies. Please don't forget that frozen yogurt, ices, ice cream, and candies can contain hidden artificial sweeteners that are offending to an enzyme-deficient patient. I find it useful during the meal to offer better and more complete coverage, particularly in situations like eating at a Mexican or Indian restaurant or dining at a restaurant that serves a salad containing vegetables, dried fruits, and offending food additives. In situations like the previous description, I use Bean-zyme along with the Digest Gold + Probiotics to ensure complete coverage.

It is important to be vigilant with your use of Bean-zyme (alpha-galactosidase), because the incidence of troublesome digestive reactions to FODMAPs is very common in the American population and occurs in people that do not necessarily present with IBS. Medical

research is needed to understand why so many people present with
this inability. Alpha-galactosidase is produced in multiple locations
in the body, and therefore we have to determine if this is due to
a reduction in alpha-galactosidase production or the development
of an inability to utilize this enzyme. No one knows for sure why
we develop this deficiency, but my theory on immune/autoimmune
reactions might be involved. This product is your best defense against
troublesome foods containing complex sugars.

It is important that you embrace the generous use of Bean-zyme.
When in doubt, always dose generously, as this ERT is relatively
inexpensive compared to Digest Gold + Probiotics, which is a full-
spectrum ERT. Digest Gold + Probiotics should be used during
your meals, during snack times, and during afternoons while eating
fruits and other FODMAPs. Always carry a generous supply of both
products with you, along with Lactaid brand lactase replacement
tablets if you feel you are lactose intolerant.

Please be aware that due to the nature of EPIEI, or IBS, which has the
characteristics of presenting symptoms that are not always constant, can
in turn have an inconsistent effect on treatment. What I mean is that you
might take your enzyme-replacement therapy and still experience some
symptoms or discomfort. For example, you might have hyperacidity
and not treat for it with antacids, the amount of ERT capsules might
not be enough for the chosen meal, or your timing might be off. If you
did not prepare the meal or ate out, then the possibility of unknown
contents containing offending foods is a great possibility. As I said, it
is not always perfect and problem free. It is important to remember
that each patient can present with varying degrees of EPIEI's resulting
in inconsistent outcomes. Inadequate stomach acid production can
influence digestive issues. A majority of the time, this remedy works
quite well. Just remain vigilant and observant and you will learn and
understand your particular requirements that will afford you relief.

CHAPTER 10

Physician Notes and Participation

I want to be perfectly clear and honest with my intent for this book. In no way am I criticizing or chastising physicians concerning my approach to the diagnosis and treatment of IBS. It is my sincerest belief that physicians are the victims of the research, teaching, and training that they receive in medical school based on inaccurate knowledge. It is not the fault of physicians that patients for IBS encounter an arduous workup that reveals inconclusive results. Since I am not a physician, I have no credence to criticize a physician concerning IBS. I continue to maintain my respect for medicine and physicians.

My discovery was afforded to me through a a chain of events that enabled me to arrive at an etiology for IBS based on past and current published research both in veterinary medicine and human medicine. The fact that I have extensive medical knowledge and I became a lab rat afforded me the opportunity to extrapolate and correlate the data, form a hypothesis for the etiology of IBS, and develop an IBS treatment protocol. In essence I was inside, at ground zero, looking out. You could say I was internally observing the action of EPIEI (Exocrine Pancreatic Intestinal Enzyme Insufficiency) at ground level.

In my view, the physician and the patient should remain partners in the coordinated effort to treat the patient. The treatment protocol requires a patient to be compliant in order to achieve success. It is necessary, ethical, and prudent for the physician to work up the patient upon intake and complete the full workup—including blood panels, endoscopy, colonoscopy, ultrasound, and CAT scan, if so indicated—to rule out other possible etiologies. I have created a short questionnaire that I feel could be useful, and I encourage its use. There is no question about the strong evidence of autoimmune response disease as a progenitor of the development of IBS. The importance of an IBS patient maintaining a working relationship with his or her physician is vital to the success of the treatment protocol. As we are all aware, one of the greatest roadblocks to effective medical treatment outcome is noncompliance in patients. We cannot lose sight of the fact that many patients are inept when it comes to medicine, and a physician guiding the IBS patient on the institution of this new treatment protocol for IBS would be most prudent. Digest Gold + Probiotics and Bean-zyme are available to the general public. Unfortunately, products available in vitamin shops, nutrition stores, and other retail facilities carry products that contain trace amounts of enzymes required or have insufficient concentrations of the required enzyme replacements, meaning they would prove valueless to IBS sufferers.

Patient's Personal History

In addition to the standard intake forms concerning
your health and required personal information, these
questions can be useful to your physician.

1. When did you first experience your symptoms?

2. How did you achieve relief from your symptoms, if ever?

3. Have you detected what foods might cause your symptoms?

4. Do you currently have an autoimmune disease?

5. Are you a type 1 or type 2 diabetic?

6. Does your family have a history of diabetes?

7. Do you have eczema?

8. Do you have allergies?

9. Are you lactose intolerant?

10. Have you ever had a severe intense gastrointestinal infection?

11. Were you ever diagnosed with pancreatitis?

12. Do you have siblings, parents, or other family members who have IBS?

13. Do you have psoriasis?

14. Do you have lupus?

15. Do you have arthritis?

16. Do you have food allergies, such as allergies to peanuts, cherries, or other foods?

17. Is there a history of Crohn's disease in your family?

18. Is there a history of celiac disease in your family?

Irritable Bowel Syndrome (IBS) Severity Score

1. How severe has your abdominal pain been over the last ten days?
    0 1 2 3 4 5 6 7 8 9 10
    (0 = no pain, 10 = very severe pain)

2. On how many of the last ten days did you experience pain?_____

3. How severe has your abdominal distention (bloating, swelling, or tightness) been over the last ten days?
    0 1 2 3 4 5 6 7 8 9 10
    (0 = no distention, 10 = very severe distention)

4. How satisfied have you been with your bowel movements (frequency, ease, etc.) over the last ten days?
    0 1 2 3 4 5 6 7 8 9 10
    (0 = very satisfied, 10 = very unsatisfied)

5. How much has your IBS been affecting/interfering with your life in general over the last ten days?
    0 1 2 3 4 5 6 7 8 9 10
    (0 = not at all, 10 = completely)

6. How many days per week do you experience normal stools? _____

7. After an IBS episode, how many days does it take to experience a normal bowel movement? _____

8. After an episode, how many days pass before you no longer experience pain, soreness, or discomfort? _____[1]

---

[1] C. Y. Francis, J. Morris, & P. J. Whorwell, "The irritable bowel severity scoring system: a simple method of monitoring irritable bowel syndrome and its progress," *Aliment Pharmacol Ther.* 11 (1997): 395–402.

CHAPTER 11

New Treatments, Theories, and Final Points

It Is Time to Eavesdrop on a Conversation

Medical research is moving at a very rapid pace, which is yielding new discoveries, understanding, treatments, and cures. Our gut or intestinal tract is extremely complex, as you have learned throughout this book. Owing to the complexities of digestion, it is not too hard to comprehend why unknowns and lack of understanding of digestion and IBS still persists today.

This chapter is devoted to a new frontier—the brain-gut axis, the microbiome, and the microbiota within and on the surface of the body. The average person thinks that he or she is immortal, invincible, and in all likelihood superior and secure in his or her environment. What we fail to realize is that human beings have many relationships with the animal and plant kingdoms. What most patients, most physicians, and the average person do not realize is that our bodies have a much greater degree of communication between our organ systems and our immune system on a cellular level than was previously known. Most microscopic environmental relationships are symbiotic, meaning that the relationship is for the mutual benefit of two entities without causing harm to either one. Some such relationships are parasitic, and one entity derives benefits from the other at the expense of the host. Examples are parasitic organisms such as pathogenic bacteria, viruses, and protozoa such as amoebas that can cause disease.

I have previously discussed the microbiome, and I mentioned that we have an estimated ten trillion residential bacteria basically living in our intestines in a symbiotic relationship. Recent discoveries in medicine have drawn attention to this important relationship and how it affects our lives. You are likely wondering why we have ten trillion bacteria in our intestine, how they got there, and what function they serve.

Throughout this book, I emphasize the importance of exercising patience and time in dealing with IBS. The nature of Americans is to always seek a quick and easy approach in the hope of attaining a rapid resolution. I am sorry to say that you cannot employ that approach with treating IBS. We are always assuming that a physician will have a magic bullet in his or her arsenal—a little super pill that will cure what ails you. As Americans, we must change that attitude or we will not accomplish the resolutions that we seek. Just remember that it took eleven months for the brush border lining of my small intestine to regain a majority of its functionality after I adjusted my diet and commenced enzyme-replacement therapy.

As I talk about the human microbiome, you will learn about its importance and how it evolved. When we study medicine, both physiological and mental, it is useful to observe animal behavior. Humans often think that they are godlike and are above the animal kingdom, but we view animals through our eyes. In past centuries, scientists believed that dogs and other species did not think. Of course that is not true, and the real truth is that we communicate poorly with other animals. I equate that defect to the scenario of an American going to a small Chinese village and trying to communicate with the people without the ability to read or speak Chinese.

If we observe a moose and watch a newborn moose being taught by its mother how to eat, we can learn how the mother helps develop the microbiome for the newborn. The baby moose observes the mother eating berries, plants, and other fruits. The mother licks the plant leaves and fruits, depositing existing bacteria from her saliva onto the leaves. When the baby moose attempts to mimic its mother, it receives a complement of beneficial bacteria that end up populating its bacteria-free gut. So how do humans accomplish this feat? Prior to birth, humans also lack gut bacteria, and so the gut is bacteria free. As the baby passes through the birth canal, the newborn picks up the bacteria lining the birth canal. This maternal bacteria enter the newborn's oral pharynx and populate the gut and establish residence in the intestinal tract to form that symbiotic relationship.

So why are the bacteria that compose the microbiome so important, and what function do they perform? Throughout this book I make analogies to baking and its complexities. During baking, we use yeast to perform the vital function of making dough rise. Those little yeast animals normally do not harm us and aid in the action of producing gas during fermentation in order to make the dough rise. A similar action occurs in brewing beer.

Now for our ten trillion friends. In a normal gut, these ten trillion residential bacteria aid in digestion. They can metabolize our waste products from the breakdown of the components of our food. These large populations of bacteria can help keep a homeostatic balance between the good guys and bad guys, keeping the pathogenic bacteria in check and controlled. I previously discussed lactobacillus in the ilium—a bacterium that helps metabolize milk sugar in dairy products in addition to the lactase enzymes produced by the body. The bacteria that make up the microbiome are our partners in digestion.

This following quote clearly explains the vital function of your microbiome:

> Remarkably, given this high inter-individual variability in the gut microbiota composition, a core gut microbiome, shared by healthy adults, has been identified, which suggests that it plays a role in the maintenance of health status. To date, a number of functions have been associated to the core microbiome, including polysaccharide digestion, immune system development, defense against infections, synthesis of vitamins, fat storage, angiogenesis regulation, and behavior development. Interestingly, genes encoded by the human core microbiome encode proteins required for host survival, but not present in the human genome, this finding led to the definition of the microbiome as "our forgotten organ."[2]

So what is being said here? The microbiome (i.e., the normal ten trillion bacteria that reside in your intestine) performs several vital functions, some of which even go beyond the action of digestion. The average person thinks that he or she is bacteria free unless he or she succumbs to illness, but of course that is just not true. We live in both a macro and micro world, and that means that although we live with all the other members of the animal kingdom, which comprises people, farm animals, pets, etc., we also live with microscopic members that make up the micro world. The average person never thinks about the bacteria living naturally on the surface of his or her skin and in

---

[2] Valeria D'Argento, Francesco Salvatore, "The role of the gut microbiome in the healthy adult status," published by B. V. Elsevier. This is an open access article under the CC BY-NC-ND license. https://www.researchgate.net/publication/270909805_The_role_of_the_gut_microbiome_in_the_healthy_adult_status.

his or her nasal passages, intestines, and other systems. The varied microorganisms within and on the surface of the body normally live in a symbiotic relationship with the human body. I will discuss why existing bacteria that are pathogens living on and within human beings usually do not present a threat but yet sometimes become virulent enough to cause disease.

We do indeed take microorganisms for granted, but they perform vital functions in our lives. They assist us in food production, such as fermentation in the production of wine and beer. They assist in cheese making and the baking of breads and cakes. This discussion will deal with two aspects of the microbiome: the understanding of what the composition of the microbiome is, and the unique communication abilities that exist on a cellular level and how the brain is directly involved in communication throughout the digestive system and actually all of the other systems of the body.

When we address the issues of IBS, we cannot ignore the ten trillion residents that exist within the gut of each of us, as they exert multiple influences on our bodies. After reading the previous quotation, you can see that your microbiome bacteria members aid in vitamin processing and absorption, which is vital to our health. What stands out in that quotation is our microbiome bacteria's involvement in polysaccharide digestion, immune system development, defense against infections, and synthesis of vitamins. The IBS sufferer should clearly see the word "polysaccharide" as a flashing warning light in addition to understanding vitamin deficiencies.

Those sugars—polysaccharides—cause us massive problems if we have compromised brush borders or exocrine pancreas cells. Simply put, some members of your microbiome can and will process and ferment those polysaccharide sugars in an out-of-control fashion when you are enzyme deficient, in turn yielding gas, bloating, cramps, and pain.

Without beating a dead horse, I will simply note that by now you certainly understand what IBS is and how your symptoms develop. Now it is time to note some shocking new discoveries and developments in twenty-first-century medicine. I will now discuss your nervous system. When you finish this book, you will have a better working knowledge and comprehension of human anatomy, digestion, and functioning of the human body.

The Brain-Gut Axis

I have said numerous times that we take our bodies and lives for granted, but the brain and nervous system win the top prize. As much as you think that you control all that goes on in your life, think again. The largest organ in your body is your skin, but one of the largest organs is your brain. That four-pound gray organ in your head is more complex and more powerful than a combined total of more than one thousand existing advanced computers. Your nervous system is the master and controller of all. Your brain communicates with every system and cell in your body. Neurology is by far the last frontier on the macro and micro levels. Can you conceive that a thought you create can actually be stored within cells in your brain in a complex chemical action, while computers store and process information digitally in series of zeros and ones? So how does your brain do it?

Obviously we have not cracked that code as of yet, but the storage and transmission of information throughout your body is more than likely accomplished via integrated chemical and electrical circuits and actions. All throughout this book, you have been thinking about why the action of digestion is so complex and convoluted, and now we are adding the brain into the mix, but it is an integral part of digestion. Think for a moment about a stressful situation in your life (e.g., taking a test when you were a student, going to a job interview, going on a first date, or being stressed about trying to pay bills when you are short on money). Of course you know exactly what I mean because you have had stomachaches, butterflies in your stomach, and all of the other reactions to stress.

Think of your body as a high-rise building. The building has a complex massive electrical grid and a system that powers every component. In the basement of that building is the "brain," which controls the heating, cooling, telephone, lighting, plumbing, transportation (elevators and escalators), and Internet. The building's brain is a computer, usually located in the basement, that is connected to every single system via electrical wiring, just like the neurological system of your body. At the entry source of the building is a large trunk cable that brings the electrical source to the building. This cable is in turn connected to smaller wires with smaller diameters for electric sockets, light switches, and other end circuts. Your body has large nerves that emanate from your brain that are part of a massive system of nerves throughout your body. The nervous system is similar to the electrical system of the building because it has nerves of varying diameters that communicate with the master, or brain. You have microscopic nerve endings in your skin and, for that matter, in the mucosal lining of your small intestine that facilitates the two-way conversation between their surrounding environment and the brain.

I will not go into heavy anatomy or neurology, but I will just say that we have two neurological systems in our bodies called the sympathetic and parasympathetic nervous systems. There is a large nerve that runs from your brain; this is called the vagus nerve. Just like a telephone wire, this nerve carries two-way transmissions between your brain and intestine, and that is why the term "brain-gut axis" was coined. Those conversations can originate from either side of the system.

To complicate matters, we are discovering that certain cells of the body can communicate with neurons (nerve cells). Research has been done by Robert Spengler, PhD, and Tracey A. Ignatowski, PhD, on how macrophages can communicate with neurons. Why is this so important? The macrophages are your disease fighters and members of your immune system. Remember that the brain has a two-way communication channel with your gut, so your brain can receive a signal from the neurons in the mucosal lining of your intestines, which receive communications from the macrophages telling the brain of troublesome situations in your gut. The reverse can be true too. A psychiatric disorder can influence an IBS response. The brain can alter cellular action via electrical transmission of messages from the brain to your gut. We know that depression can present with an inflammatory response in the brain. Think about the famous sayings "Mind over matter" and "If you don't mind, then it doesn't matter." The idea of being mentally strong or weak can influence the body, and the brain can certainly influence the state of your gut.

The immune system is responsible for producing inflammation, which can directly affect IBS. I have discussed inflammation before, and one issue regarding it is uncontrolled inflammation. Your brain can initiate an inflammatory response in the gut to mental stress just as easily as the presence of a pathogen can marshal a response from a macrophage because of its presence. Of course you know this is true. When you get a stomach virus or other GI infection, how do you become aware of the changes? The brain-gut axis communicates the state of your gut, of course.

Remember that IBS is a condition that has a broad array of etiologies (causes). Medicine is not at the stage of developing a pharmaceutical that you will take three times per day for two weeks and become cured. My entire approach to IBS in this book relates to treating the symptoms and not curing the broad spectrum of etiologies. Now that you understand how my own personal IBS condition evolved, you can understand that one of the most important approaches to an effective resolution is exercising patience. It took eleven months for me to achieve a reasonably reconstructed and functioning brush border.

An easy analogy for understanding my approach is to look at what happens when you sustain a temporary injury. Under normal conditions, your body repairs the damage and you recover. Think about what happens when a person receives repeated blows, such as head trauma resulting in concussions and traumatic brain injuries. After repeated physical trauma, your body can become so overwhelmed, and your brain so compromised, that you cannot return to normal. What happens if you repeatedly receive abrasions and a deep bruises to your elbow? At some point in time, your elbow will not fully recover; and in addition to massive scarring, you might in fact sustain permanent joint damage. Simply put, I theorize that my out-of-control immune system resulting from my chemotherapy inflicted permanent damage to my brush border. The fact that I am predisposed to autoimmune disease poses the questions of whether I was a candidate to start GM-CSF or Leukine and whether I should have engaged in that anticancer treatment therapy.

You can see that the situation is very complex; I just wanted to give you a brief overview of how your brain interacts with your gut.

Following are a few new attempts at novel treatment for EPIEI or IBS.

- **Probiotics**: Probiotic treatment is based on the idea of trying to reintroduce friendly bacteria colonies into the gut or intestine to help achieve hemostasis and a better balance of bacterial species within the gut. Unfortunately, in my view, this will not achieve success because of the presence of virulent pathogens and undigested complex sugars in the small intestine. In certain instances it can be beneficial, but I sincerely doubt that it will offer relief for those who are exocrine pancreatic enzyme insufficient or intestinal enzyme insufficient. Probiotics cannot always be delivered to the relevant region of the guttube.

- **Fecal Microbiota Transplant (FMT):** This is a newly developed procedure that is exactly what the title implies. The theory and impetus here is to take a fecal donor sample from a patient that does not present with IBS or other digestive or gastrointestinal issues and transplant the sample into the recipient's colon. It is believed that this recolonizes the good bacteria in an attempt to achieve homeostasis. In my opinion, this procedure can work in certain individuals; however, those who present with EPIEI most likely will not benefit, owing to the continued presence of complex sugars that have not been broken down. Naturally the complex sugar food source will continue to stimulate the propagation of excessive bacterial populations along with a percentage of virulent species that will cause the immune system to produce an inflammatory response.

- **Antidepressants:** Some gastroenterologists have been prescribing these medications in an attempt to help reduce the symptoms of IBS. Naturally some believe that IBS can be caused by psychosomatic issues, and so there has been minor success with such treatments. This is an important consideration, as your digestive tract is one of the largest organs in the body that contains vast amounts of sensory receptors. After all, its composition is similar in nature to that of your skin. Its origins are the same (i.e., epithelial cells). The surface area of your digestive lining is about 344 square feet, and there are extensive sensory nerve endings in the lining of your gut that sense changes in all that passes over them. Those sensory nerve endings send signals to the vagus nerve, which communicates directly with your brain. Hence, when you feel pain, discomfort, soreness, and other discomforts, those feelings are sent directly to your brain. Use of antipsychotics can be an adjunct to treating certain aspects of IBS. This is discussed in greater detail in the previous discussion of the brain-gut axis.

- **Steroidal Treatment**: All too often, steroids are used as a last resort or as an option when no other treatment seems to offer relief. The purpose of prescribing steroids for the treatment of IBS is to attempt to reduce inflammation. Remember that a resultant inflammatory response is an immune action and a reaction to a pathogen (bacteria, virus) or an insult to the mucosal lining of your gut. Steroids treat the symptoms and not the cause. Long-term use of steroids can have many resultant side effects that can cause damage to a patient. The risks far outweigh the temporary relief steroids can achieve. In a diabetic patient, steroids can play havoc with blood sugar and promote elevated blood sugars.

- **Xifaxan**: I discussed this new antibiotic previously in this book. The FDA just approved Xifaxan in May, 2015, for the treatment of IBS-D (IBS that presents with diarrhea). You already know that this is futile and unnecessary.

Fecal Production and Formation

This subject is mostly overlooked and never discussed because of embarrassment or distaste for the subject matter. However, this is part of a normal process of digestion that mostly occurs each day but is usually ignored in a discussion with the patient's physician. Acceptance of the average person's fecal state—whether it be normal, loose, frequent, oddly shaped, firm, hard, small, large, buoyant, or otherwise different from what is considered average—is usually ignored. The state of one's bowel movement—its shape, consistency, and composition—is a true window into the physiology and condition of the person's digestive system.

The composition of stool is approximately 30 percent water, 30 percent undigested food, fiber, and waste by-products, and 30 percent bacteria, and the balance contains some protein and fat. In normal people, by the time digested food arrives in the colon or large intestine, the body has already absorbed the nutrients from the chyme. The main function of the large intestine is water and salt reclamation. The physical state of the feces can reflect the degree of completion of digestion and food or nutrient absorption that occurred in the small intestine. Remember that if a person's brush border is compromised or damaged, then food absorption and digestion can be hampered and reduced owing to the lack of digestive enzymes from a deficient exocrine pancreas or reduced enterocyte enzyme-producing cells on the brush border villi.

The key here is the physical condition and state of the brush border, which I have previously discussed. If your brush border is compromised and not functioning normally, then IBS issues can develop. IBS issues can arise from breaks in the latticework of the structure of the brush border due to damage to the enterocyte cell latticework and the mucosal lining. If there are breaks in the brush border, you can develop what is described as a leaky gut. Fluid can enter the gut, which can cause increased water concentration in the feces or stool, which in turn can contribute to the development of diarrhea. The osmotic pressure can be affected by the degree of permeability. This means that if there are breaks in the brush border—which normally functions as the gatekeeper for protecting the body by keeping pathogenic bacteria from exiting the intestine and moving into the surrounding tissues by maintaining a tight, single-celled layer—then it becomes a two-way path. Your stool's consistency can reflect improper digestion, increased amounts of pathogenic bacteria, increased amounts of undigested or un-metabolized sugars, and possibly fats.

Trouble Shooting Guide

Throughout this book I have been very clear in reinforcing that my treatment modality is not a cure but a treatment. Remember that there will be incidents when you experience a reoccurrence of your previous symptoms (e.g., sharp abdominal pain, gas, bloating, lose stools, and frequent bowel movements). Because of the nature of EPIEI or IBS, the varying degrees of symptoms and frequency are self-evident. The following are hints to help you understand why you might have encountered an episode of discomfort or a gastrointestinal incident.

Possible Reasons for an Occurrence

Remember that the greatest offending foods are garlic and onions, along with the others on the top of the FODMAP list.

- You had hyperacidity when you took your ERT (Enzyme Replacement Therapy) and you failed to take an antacid to prevent the destruction of the enzymes when they entered your stomach.
- You failed to take enough ERT before your meal.
- Your meal had higher concentrations of offending foods then you anticipated.
- The type of meal you had consisted of multiple offending foods spread throughout several courses that required additional ERT capsules during the meal, and you failed to compensate accordingly. (Remember that you can open the capsule and sprinkle the contents directly on the food to enhance coverage if needed.)
- You ate a snack and thought that because it was small you didn't need to take your ERT.

- You ate out at a restaurant or at someone's home and didn't take extra ERT to cover yourself against unknown ingredients in the meal.
- Restaurants often spray their prepared dishes with butter for a shiny, juicy look.
- Even though the meal appeared to be foods that are not offending, you failed to consider unknown ingredients in salad dressings, sauces, and toppings.
- You failed to ask if a food had been cooked in butter.

Remember to always approach any anticipated meal by over supplementing rather than acting conservatively by dispensing less ERT. Excess ingestion of digestive enzymes will not harm you; the enzymes will just be metabolized or digested.

CONCLUSION

All of the people who are involved in and connected to medicine share one common goal, and that is to facilitate the reduction and alleviation of pain and suffering in our society. The phrases "the art of medicine" and "the practice of medicine" show that medicine encompasses much more than the patient realizes. The degree of artistic ability in practicing medicine can dictate how good a diagnostician the physician can be. Medicine is not an exact science, in that a physician cannot predict an accurate response to a medication or predict how long it will take for a patient to recover from an infection, operation, or other crisis. Physicians respond based on average responses to a pathogen, medication, and medical intervention. The reason for this is that they are dealing with the human body. Each patient presents with his or her own unique body's genetic complement, which can effect different responses to stressors presented by pathogens, environmental issues, toxins, metabolic anomalies, psychological stressors, and other insults to our bodies.

The age-old question is, why are there variances, and why does uniformity not exist in human beings? Of course the answer is that we are all different because of each individual's own unique genetic makeup. Even though human beings receive twenty-three chromosomes from each parent, the human zygote produced after the union of the sperm and ovum is not a carbon copy of either parent. That new zygote is a mixture of genes from both parents. It is extremely complex, but what we are dealing with is genetics. I discuss this because this action created a unique you. This can influence how you might react to environmental influences and the effect of the microbiome.

What I am saying here is that not all genes that have been inherited and formulated are perfect or positive in kind. The term "polymorphism" describes the variation and deviation in genetics that can be expressed in variations of a specific gene. Even though a person inherits a gene, it can, in fact, be a deviation of that gene. As you are likely well aware, deviant genes can be responsible for disease and medical conditions such as diabetes, MS, ALS, and others on the long list of inherited genetic disorders. The presence of polymorphism can even affect the way an individual responds to medications. In relation to IBS or EPIEI, there is no question that autoimmunity plays a major role here. As we progress in this century, we will discover that more diseases have origins in autoimmune response actions than most people realize.

In this regard, we must realize that medicine is currently attempting to treat the symptoms of IBS and not the cause. Even though we already know that type 1 diabetes is an autoimmune response disease, we currently have not been able to avert its development. Those who are genetically predisposed for the disease have not been able to prevent it. All attempts to date have been unsuccessful in averting a full-blown case of type 1 diabetes by preventing destruction of beta cells—the insulin-producing cells within the pancreas. As we discussed previously, the development of type 2 diabetes can be averted in a majority of cases by controlling weight gain and adhering to a specific diet.

I used the term "diverse" in relation to reaction to disease, and that term truly describes IBS because it presents with varying degrees of severity and symptoms. Nonetheless, my treatment protocol is an effective treatment for most cases, provided the patient consciously remains observant of his or her intake of all foods and medicates accordingly. The unfortunate caveat here is that the patient is, in fact, treating the symptoms and not the cause, even though the causative agent is presumably the immune system. It is my firm belief that through stem cell treatment we will one day be able to replace the destroyed and nonexistent brush border enzyme-producing cells with new functioning ones, along with replacement pancreatic acinar cells and even beta cells in the endocrine pancreas. Remember that the brush border can be destroyed by pathogens adhering to the enterocyte cells that make up the brush border. In normal situations, your body prevents this action. It is believed that intestinal alkaline phosphatase (IAP) prevents the adherence of pathogenic bacteria to the brush border enterocyte cells, and so if a patient has a reduction or absence of IAP, then his or her brush border might sustain damage from a pathogenic bacterium.

Medicine is a very rigid profession that yields very slowly to new ideas and change. Physicians need the ability to think outside the box, and this is the key to being a good diagnostician. Not all patients with a suspected condition or illness present the same. In addition, the resultant condition might not have just a single etiology and might in fact be more than one condition or suspected disease. Often a patient presents with a bacterial and a viral infection concurrently. To add to that scenario, the patient could end up with a fungal infection due to excessive antibiotic treatment. So what appears to be the obvious is not always necessarily true.

When we consider the broad scope of IBS, its diverse symptoms, and the lack of resolution attained in current treatment approaches, it makes one wonder how this could be so prevalent in medicine today. It is very easy to postulate theories and offer remedies hawked on the

Internet that have no supportive research to back up their claims. But when you observe how many sites there are for IBS, it makes you realize how prevalent this disorder is in our population. Why are my theories correct? Simple: the treatment has successfully resolved my IBS, provided I remain on the treatment protocol. This was an A-B-A trial treatment (Applied Behavior Analysis). Why was I able to figure out the etiology of IBS when others couldn't? You read the answer in this book. In essence I induced major insults to my body via the use of chemotherapy, GM-CSF, which grossly heightened my immune system. I became the lab rat in my research and I developed IBS in the same fashion as we induce diseases or medical conditions in lab mice or canines such as inducing type 1 diabetes and other disorders in order to study the same.

There is one other consideration. When a person is suffering from a medical condition, in most situations he or she tends to discuss his or her condition with those who have the same condition. I personally encountered countless people who have IBS or EPIEI, as well as friends and family members of those who have the disorder. They all exhibit similar symptoms in varying degrees of severity, and they all complain about their inability to achieve relief or resolve of their IBS.

I leave you with the most important advice and a word of caution. Please be well aware that I am not a medical researcher and do not possess a PhD; nor am I a physician. All through my adult life I have had a love and passion for medicine, and I majored in pre-medicine during my time in university. Throughout my life, I followed medicine and always stayed up to date on the latest medical discoveries, theories, and new procedures. Aside from my love for medicine, I found it necessary to stay well educated in medicine because I was a type 1 diabetic. I knew early on that education was the best defense against the complications that arise from diabetes. I employed the same technique to combat my IBS or EPIEI.

I implore you to be patient and vigilant with the program that I have laid out for you in this book. It is of utmost importance that you do not expect a rapid and accelerated improvement in a few days. Do not confuse this treatment with that of being on a round of antibiotics for a streptococcus infection. The repair process of reestablishing an intact mucosal lining of your gut takes *time*. I implore you to exercise *patience*. If you do, you will achieve positive results. Remember that every patient is different in terms of damage and in terms of which EPIEs are deficient. Also bear in mind that I am not prescribing medicine. I am, however, educating you on digestion and digestive enzyme insufficiencies that can be corrected via ERT (Enzyme Replacement Therapy).

This program has worked for me, has restored normalcy to my life, and has reduced most of my suffering. You will accomplish the same if you stay the course. Remember that it took almost one year for me to attain fair recovery. Think back to a time when you sustained a bad gastrointestinal viral or bacterial infection. How long did it take for your mucosal lining to heal and return to normal? How long was it before you embraced normal eating or even made attempts at gluttony? Now magnify that time frame tenfold or more and you can understand the complexities of the repair process and the necessity of time that your gut needs to achieve reasonable resolution.

During your approach to achieving a resolution or improvement of your IBS, I implore you to exercise patience and vigilance. Remember that you are at the mercy of your own body's ability to start and progress in the rebuilding process of your brush border—the lining of your small intestine. My theory is based on understanding celiac disease and what occurs in this genetically predisposed disease. It is an extreme version of what can occur in IBS in terms of symptoms but involves excessive and total gluten intolerance. Understand that medical science extensively studied celiac disease and zeroed in on its etiology and what resultant damage occurs in a celiac disease patient. I bring this up again because of the time required to facilitate the repair process of the brush border after cessation of consuming gluten.

Extensive studies were done on celiac disease that clearly showed and determined that after one year of a gluten-free diet, the patients displayed on average a 50 to 70 percent reconstructed brush border. Some patients achieved a 70 percent rebuild only after five years of being gluten free. These results beg for a clearer understanding of the physical structure and latticework formation of the brush border on a cellular level. I have mentioned several times that this is ground zero for digestion issues. Matthew Tyska, PhD, has been a prolific publisher of extensive papers at Vanderbilt University on his research of the brush border. Papers as recent as 2015 and even 2016 clearly reflect results of his research on how pathogenic bacteria compromise the brush border. This is the holy grail and the keystone to understanding IBS, and few physicians are aware or even understand these new monumental discoveries. Understanding Dr. Tyska's work and discoveries will aid the patient and the physician in developing an effective treatment plan. The key is the required time it takes for the rebuilding process of your brush border after alleviating the offending food to facilitate the repair processes.

For a clearer understanding, if you are a physician or if you have an understanding of science and medicine, then read "Brush Border Destruction by Enterohemorrhagic Escheria Coli (EHEC): New Insights From Organoid Culture," published by Matthew Tyska in January 2016.

I can now clearly state my theory on the etiology of IBS:

IBS is a condition that results from the destruction of or damage to the brush border of the small intestinal mucosal lining, which in turn compromises the body's ability to produce the necessary digestive enzymes for normal food digestion. This destructive action is due to an immunological response to a pathogenic infection. In addition, the same pathogenic inducers can translate to insufficient exocrine pancreatic enzyme production. The deficient enzymes facilitate exponential small intestinal bacterial overgrowth (SIBO).

Unfortunately, research and science are often complex and do not always yield easy and simple explanations in order to satisfy theories. As I have discussed all throughout this book, IBS is complex, and the fact that IBS has many etiologies has delayed research and development of effective treatment. The fact that I am not a physician or researcher has placed limits on my ability to improve medicine's approach to treatment of IBS. I present with IBS, and my having spent almost two years researching past case histories, my analysis of my own condition, my study of veterinary medicine's approach to pancreatitis, and my understanding of medicine all helped me to formulate my theory and treatment.

I truly believe that my etiological description of IBS, IBD, and even ulcerative colitis (UC) is the root cause and is mainly based on the presence of a compromised or destroyed brush border, which mostly occurs in the duodenum and can involve the jejunum and ilium. The reason why it becomes chronic and intermittent is because the brush border never fully repairs itself and the villi never return to their original uniform height and design. This results in damaged and or destroyed glandular enzyme-producing enterocyte cells that lack the ability to supply digestive enzymes or can supply only reduced amounts of enzymes.

Now that you have a full working knowledge of IBS you can understand why IBS is BS and should be renamed DED (digestive enzyme deficiency).

The simply stated fact about the compromised brush border, in my view, is a logical explanation for the varying degrees of IBS, UC, and IBD. Remember: not everyone has the same degree of lactose intolerance or symptoms of IBS. Therefore, at this juncture, we do not have a cure. Rather, we have a remedy, and that is broad-spectrum enzyme-replacement therapy. It is broad-spectrum treatment in that it supplies all of the required digestive enzymes—both exocrine pancreatic enzymes and brush border enzymes—because currently there are no relevant diagnostic tests available for determining enzyme deficiencies in the body.

Two years ago, I postulated that pathogens, or disease-causing bacteria and viruses, cause the demise of enzyme-producing cells in the pancreas and small intestine, and now two research papers published results from clinical research on animals that substantiate my hypothesis. I discussed this previously in this book, and the research was reported in September 2015 and February 2016.

I further believe that an additional reason certain individuals develop damage to their brush border is a genetic predisposition that compromises the person's ability to produce IAP. This chemical is produced in the brush border enterocyte glandular cells and in the liver. It protects the brush border by preventing pathogenic bacteria and viruses from adhering to the cells of the brush border, where they would be able to destroy the enterocyte cells if they adhered to them.

As for the exocrine pancreas, I have previously noted that it is known that autoimmunity causes type 1 diabetes) by destroying the beta cells in the pancreas that produce insulin. I surmise that this same action can cause destruction to the exocrine pancreatic enzyme-producing cells.

You now know and understand how a person can develop IBD and IBS.

In support of my theory, Rockefeller University just released research in February 2016 that confirms my theory on how disease and infections can cause damage to the small intestine's brush border lining. In addition, this research relates to the actions of the macrophages and how they communicate with neurons. This work is also a reaffirmation of previous original work done by Robert Spengler, PhD, and Tracey A. Ignatowski, PhD, which demonstrated the ability of macrophages to communicate with neurons.

As I previously stated, an exaggerated inflammatory response to a pathogen can not only cause damage to surrounding tissue at the site of the pathogen attack but can also go on to inflict permanent damage, as in the cases of IBS, IBD, and even CD (Crohn's disease). I implore those sufferers of UC, Crohn's disease, and IBD who are facing surgical intervention in several months' time to follow my treatment protocol to the letter for a minimum of nine months before opting for surgery, in order to see if they can initiate a brush border healing and rebuilding process. The final decision should be made only after patients discuss this with their doctors and receive approval. Hyperbaric Oxygen Therapy can be invaluable in stabilizing health and healing in some of these cases.

In view of the two above-referenced researchers, we see the confirmation of the brain-gut axis and the new discoveries of how our immune system (macrophages) communicates with nearby neurons that in turn carry on two-way conversations between the brain and gut. It is totally logical that the treatment protocol that has been discussed in this book has broad positive implications for treatment resolve in UC, IBD, and CD (Crohn's disease), in addition to IBS abatement.

It is still my firm belief that autoimmune disease plays a role in many aspects of this damaging disease action that yields IBS. It is important to realize that I myself represent an extreme case of IBS, but because of my exaggerated autoimmune response to a pathogen(s) from the chemotherapy (GM-CSF) action, it is clear that the average IBS patient should not respond to an infection to the degree that I did and can have an even greater successful outcome with the stated treatment protocol in this book.

In closing, I can clearly state that during the last eleven months of my life I have restored my life to a relatively normally functioning life after suffering IBS for fifteen years. Remember that I have not presented a cure here but a remedy. Yes, I have experienced IBS episodes, and I was able to isolate the reasons, which were (1) not compensating for hyperacidity, which nullified the enzyme-replacement therapy for the meal, (2) not taking enough enzyme replacement for the meal, or (3) ingesting an excessive amount of an offending food. I invite and encourage you to return your life to one of normalcy.

BIBLIOGRAPHY

Andren-Sandberg, Ake, and Philip D. Hardt. "Second Giessen International Workshop on Interactions of Exocrine and Endocrine Pancreatic Diseases." *Journal of the Pancreas* 9, no.4 (July 2008): 541–75.

Andriulli, Angelo, Antonio Massimo Ippolito, Virginia Festa, Maria Rosa Valvano, Antonio Merla, Fabrizio Bossa, Grazia Niro, Grazia Napolitano, Luigi Benini, and Italo Vantini. "Exocrine Pancreatic Insufficiency, as Assessed by Fecal Elastase-1 Levels, in Diabetic Patients: An Estimate of Prevalence in Prospective Studies." *J Diabetes Metab* 5 (May 30, 2014): 379. Accessed May 27, 2014. doi:10.4172/2155-6156.1000379.

Clark, L. A., J. M. Wahl, J. M. Steiner, W. Zhou, J. Wan, T. R.. Famula, D. A. Williams and K. E. Murphy. "Linkage analysis and gene expression profile of pancreatic acinar atrophy in the German Shepherd Dog." *Mammalian Genome* 16, no. 12 (December 2005): 955–62.

Clin Exp Gastroenterol. 2011; 4: 55–73. Published online 2011 May 4. doi: 10.2147/CEG.S17634 PMCID: PMC3132852 Enzyme replacement therapy for pancreatic insufficiency: present and future Aaron Fieker,1 Jessica Philpott,1 and Martine Armand2 Cummings. M. "Pancreatic exocrine insufficiency in type 1 and type 2 diabetes – more common than you think?" *Journal of Diabetes Nursing* 18 (2014): 320–3.

Di Pierro, Francesco, Alexander Bertuccioli, Eleonora Marini, and Leandro Ivaldi. "A pilot trial on subjects with lactose and/or oligosaccharides intolerance treated with a fixed mixture of pure and enteric-coated α- and β-galactosidase." *Clin Exp Gastroenterol* 8 (February 19, 2015): 95–100. doi: 10.2147/CEG.S79449.

Ewald, N. and R. G. Bretzel "Diabetes mellitus secondary to pancreatic diseases (Type 3c)--are we neglecting an important disease?" *Eur J Intern Med* 24, no. 3 (April 2013):203–6. doi: 10.1016/j.ejim.2012.12.017. Epub Feb 1, 2013.

Ewald, Nils, and Philip D. Hardt. "Diagnosis and treatment of diabetes mellitus in chronic pancreatitis." *World J Gastroenterol* 19, no. 42 (November 14, 2013): 7276–81. Published online November 14, 2013. doi: 10.3748/wjg.v19.i42.7276.

Ewald, Nils, and Philip D. Hardt. "Diagnosis and treatment of diabetes mellitus in chronic pancreatitis" *World J Gastroenterol.* 19, no. 42 (Nov 14, 2013): 7276–81. doi: 10.3748/wjg.v19.i42.7276.

Ewald, Nils, and Philip D. Hardt "Alterations in exocrine pancreatic function in diabetes mellitus." *Pancreapedia: Exocrine Pancreas Knowledge Base,* doi: 10.3998/panc.2015.7.

Fieker, Aaron, Jessica Philpott, and Martine Armand. "Enzyme replacement therapy for pancreatic insufficiency: present and future" *Clin Exp Gastroenterol* 4 (2011): 55–73. doi: 10.2147/CEG.S17634.

Gabanyi, Ilana, Paul A. Muller, Linda Feighery, Thiago Y. Oliveira, Frederico A. Costa-Pinto, and Daniel Mucida. "Neuro-immune Interactions Drive Tissue Programming in Intestinal Macrophages." *Cell* 164, no. 3 (January 28, 2016): 378–91.

Galli G1, Esposito G, Lahner E, Pilozzi E, Corleto VD, Di Giulio E, Aloe Spiriti MA, Annibale B. Department of Digestive and Liver Disease, Sant'Andrea Hospital, Sapienza University Rome, Rome, Italy. 2014 Sep;40(6):639-47. doi: 10.1111/apt.12893. Epub 2014 Jul 28. Histological recovery and gluten-free diet adherence: a prospective 1-year follow-up study of adult patients with coeliac disease.

Helander, Herbert F., Lars Fändriks. "Surface area of the digestive tract— Revisited." *Scandinavian Journal of Gastroenterology* 49, no. 6 (April 2014;). doi: 10.3109/00365521.2014.898326.

Kanth, Ravi, and D. Nageshwar Reddy. "Genetics of acute and chronic pancreatitis: An update." *World J Gastrointest Pathophysiol* 5, no. 4, (Nov 15, 2014): 427–437. doi: 10.4291/wjgp.v5.i4.427.

Le Barz, Mélanie, Fernando F. Anhê, Thibaut V. Varin, Yves Desjardins, Emile Levy, Denis Roy, Maria C. Urdaci, André Marette. "Probiotics as Complementary Treatment for Metabolic Disorders." *Diabetes Metab J* 39 (2015): 291–303 http://dx.doi.org/10.4093/dmj.2015.39.4.291.

Moayyedi, Paul, Michael G. Surette, Peter T. Kim, Josie Libertucci, Melanie Wolfe, Catherine Onischi, David Armstrong, et al. "Fecal Microbiota Transplantation Induces Remission in Patients With Active Ulcerative Colitis in a Randomized Controlled Trial." *Gastroenterology* 149 (2015): 102–9.

Neuroscience. 1994 Apr;59(4):939-52. Cholecystokinin corticostriatal pathway in the rat: evidence for bilateral origin from medial prefrontal cortical areas.Morino P1, Mascagni F, McDonald A, Hökfelt T.Oriach, C. S., R. C. Robertson, C. Stanton, J. F. Cryan, and T. G. Dinan. "Food for thought: The role of nutrition in the microbiota-gut- brain axis." *Clinical Nutrition Experimental* 6 (2016): 25–38. doi: 10.1016/ j.yclnex.2016.01.003

Ramasamy, S., D. D. Nguyen, M. A. Eston, S. N. Alam, A. K. Moss, F. Ebrahimi, B. Biswas, et al. "Intestinal alkaline phosphatase has beneficial effects in mouse models of chronic colitis." *Inflamm Bowel Dis* 17, no. 2,(February 2011): 532–42. doi: 10.1002/ibd.21377.

Scott, K. G.–E., M. R. Logan, G. M. Klammer, D. A. Teoh, and A. G. Buret. "Jejunal Brush Border Microvillous Alterations in *Giardia muris*- Infected Mice: Role of T Lymphocytes and Interleukin." *Infection and Immunity* 68, no. 6 (June 2000): 3412–8.

Spengler, Robert N., Nader D. Nader, and Tracey A. Ignatowski. "Antinociception occurs with a reversal in α2-adrenoceptor regulation of TNF production by peripheral monocytes." *Eur J Pharmacol* 588, nos. 2–3 (July 7, 2008): 217–31. doi: 10.1016/j.ejphar.2008.04.043

Tony Trang, Johanna Chan, and David Y. Graham. "Pancreatic enzyme replacement therapy for pancreatic exocrine insufficiency in the 21st century." *World J Gastroenterol* 20 no. 33 (September 7, 2014): 11467–85. doi: 10.3748/wjg. v20.i33.11467.

University of Missouri. "Anatomy and Function of the Gastrointestinal Tract." Columbia, Missouri: University of Missouri Health Care. August 29, 2008.

Vujasinovic, Miroslav, Bojan Tepes, Jana Makuc, Sasa Rudolf, Jelka Zaletel, Tjasa Vidmar, Maja Seruga, Bostjan Birsa, and Jana Makuc. "Pancreatic exocrine insufficiency, diabetes mellitus and serum nutritional markers after acute pancreatitis." *World Journal of Gastroenterology* 20 no. 48 (December 2014): 18432–8. doi: 10.3748/wjg.v20.i48.18432.

Wang, Wei, Shan-Wen Chen, Jing Zhu, Shuai Zuo, Yuan-Yuan Ma, Zi-Yi Chen, Jun-Ling Zhang, et al. "Intestinal Alkaline Phosphatase Inhibits the Translocation of Bacteria of Gut-Origin in Mice with Peritonitis: Mechanism of Action." *PLoS One* 10, no. 5 (May 6, 2015). doi: 10.1371/journal.pone.0124835.

Williams, J. M., C. A. Duckworth, M. D. Burkitt, A. J. M. Watson, B. J. Campbell, and D. M. Pritchard. "Epithelial Cell Shedding and Barrier Function: A Matter of Life and Death at the Small Intestinal Villus Tip" *Veterinary Pathology* 52, no.3 (May 2015): 445–55. doi: 10.1177/0300985814559404.

Yang, Jian-Feng, Mark Fox, Hua Chu, Xia Zheng, Yan-Qin Long, Daniel Pohl, Michael Fried, and Ning Dai. "Four-sample lactose hydrogen breath test for diagnosis of lactose malabsorption in irritable bowel syndrome patients with diarrhea." *World J Gastroenterol* 21, no. 24 (June 28 2015): 7563–70.

Zhou, Xiaohui, Ramiro H. Massol, Fumihiko Nakamura, Xiang Chen, Benjamin E. Gewurz, Brigid M. Davis, Wayne I. Lencer, and Matthew K. Waldor. "Remodeling of the Intestinal Brush Border Underlies Adhesion and Virulence of an Enteric Pathogen." *mBio* 5, no. 4 (2014). doi: 10.1128/mBio.01639-14.